THE MAUDSLEY
Maudsley Monographs

MAUDSLEY MONOGRAPHS

HENRY MAUDSLEY, from whom the series of monographs takes its name, was the founder of The Maudsley Hospital and the most prominent English psychiatrist of his generation. The Maudsley Hospital was united with the Bethlem Royal Hospital in 1948 and its medical school, renamed the Institute of Psychiatry at the same time, became a constituent part of the British Postgraduate Medical Federation. It is now associated with King's College, London, and entrusted with the duty of advancing psychiatry by teaching and research. The Bethlem-Maudsley NHS Trust, together with the Institute of Psychiatry, are jointly known as The Maudsley.

The monograph series reports work carried out at The Maudsley. Some of the monographs are directly concerned with clinical problems; others, less obviously relevant, are in scientific fields that are cultivated for the furtherance of psychiatry.

Maudsley Monographs number forty

Psychosis in the inner city:
The Camberwell first episode study

David J. Castle
University of Western Australia, Perth, Western Australia

Simon Wessely
Department of Psychological Medicine, King's College School of Medicine and Dentistry, and Institute of Psychiatry, London, UK

Jim Van Os
University of Limburg, Maastricht, The Netherlands

Robin M. Murray
Department of Psychological Medicine, King's College School of Medicine and Dentistry, and Institute of Psychiatry, London, UK

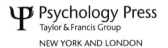

Psychology Press
Taylor & Francis Group

NEW YORK AND LONDON

Published 1998 by Psychology Press
711 Third Avenue, New York, NY 10017, USA
27 Church Road, Hove, East Sussex BN3 2FA

First issued in paperback 2014

Psychology Press is an imprint of the Taylor & Francis Group, an informa business

British Library Cataloguing in Publication Data

A catalogue record for this book is available from the British Library

ISSN 0076-5465

ISBN 13: 978-1-138-87183-0 (pbk)
ISBN 13: 978-0-86377-516-1 (hbk)

Typeset by Quorum Technical Services Ltd, Cheltenham

Contents

Acknowledgements

Many individuals contributed to the production of this book. In particular, we thank Dr Pak Sham for his guidance with the latent class and SKUMIX analyses, and Dr Robert Howard for his practical and intellectual contributions to the chapter on late-onset psychosis. Anna Waterreus collated the references, and Jenny Marchant provided ongoing support and assistance. DC acknowledges the support of the Medical Research Council, and SW of the Wellcome Trust. The vision of Professor John Wing in establishing the Camberwell Register should also be acknowledged.

We would like to thank the publishers of the following journals for their kind permission to reproduce copyrighted material in this book. They include: *British Journal of Psychiatry*; *International Journal of Geriatric Psychiatry*; *Psychological Medicine* and *Schizophrenia Bulletin*.

Preface

Notwithstanding all the advances in general knowledge about the human brain and behaviour, and the tremendous potential of our research technologies, schizophrenia in the late 1990s remains as enigmatic as dementia praecox was in the late 1890s. Understandably, the expectation is high that the key to causation will be found by biological research, and that a major breakthrough in unravelling susceptibility genes or a specific cellular or neurochemical pathology in schizophrenia is inevitable—*vide* Huntington or Alzheimer disease. However, a critical examination of the premises on which such success would be achievable in the instance of schizophrenia gives less reason for unqualified optimism. First, the disease entity of schizophrenia is a working hypothesis which has not been strictly and unequivocally validated. Second, even under the assumption that it is an hypothetical entity, agreement is lacking on its divisibility—one syndrome or many? Third, its boundaries towards the affective disorders on one hand, and towards schizoid or schizotypal personality variants on the other hand, remain in dispute. If such basic problems stay unresolved, by confounding the questions, they will continue to undermine the capacity of the biological research techniques to provide the answers.

Epidemiology has a vital role to play in this respect by exploring the attributes of the clinical concept of schizophrenia and their correlates in relation to the population base from which cases are dawn. Although many clinical and biological studies still operate with truncated distributions of such attributes because of unsystematic or opportunity sampling, an epidemiological sample is less likely to be affected by such bias and more likely to be representative of the entire spectrum of manifestations of the notional disease. The study of epidemiologically defined samples of schizophrenia cases should therefore lead to more precise questions about syndrome boundaries, clinical heterogeneity, and associations with possible risk factors.

Opportunities for such studies are relatively rare, and this underscores the value of the monograph by Castle, Wessely, Van Os and Murray. It is based on a case notes review of 486 verified cases of "non-affective psychoses" (86% of the total) who made a first-ever contact with services reporting to the Camberwell Register (now regrettably defunct) during 1965–1984. Notably, the recording of first contacts, rather than first admissions, revealed that, on average, 20% of all patients with schizophrenia are not hospitalised during the first illness episode. If this incidental finding reflects a widespread trend in the management of psychotic illness, it may have a bearing on the contentious issue of a declining incidence of schizophrenia in certain parts of the world.

A special merit of the study is that all cases received a research diagnosis through a standardised scoring procedure using the OPCRIT polydiagnostic algorithm, which reduced substantially the diagnostic variation inherent in hospital records. Having thus established an epidemiologically anchored clinical database, the authors proceed to address a number of "hot spot" issues in schizophrenia research: the relationships between gender, age at onset and syndromal characteristics of the disorder; the description of late onset schizophrenia; criminal behaviour and schizophrenia; stability of incidence rates over time; and the incidence of psychotic illness in ethnic minorities. In addition, the authors have addressed the question of the short-term prognosis of schizophrenia by a 4-year 'follow-back' study of 153 patients who had an onset of psychotic illness within the previous 5 years.

To mention some of the highlights of the monograph, the analyses of crime and schizophrenia, and of the comparative incidence of disorders in African-Caribbean and African immigrants, are methodologically ingenious and lead to well supported conclusions. The description of the clinical profile of late-onset schizophrenia is a timely contribution to a topic which attracts less attention in the current literature than is warranted by its critical importance for any aetiological theories about the disorder. The discussion of the complex issue of gender differences in the incidence, clinical manifestations and short-term outcome is less conclusive but it clearly points to questions that need to be addressed by further research.

It is up to the reader to pick up themes for reflection and further inquiry from this richly documented monograph. Among the many issues discussed, I find two which are particularly challenging. The first is the "goodness of fit" between the epidemiological data reported here and the bulk of evidence from other research which, in the absence of any strong evidence to the contrary, suggests that the incidence of schizophrenia is comparable across different populations and stable across time periods. This uniformity sets schizophrenia apart from many other disorders and has no straightforward explanation. However, there is strong evidence that schizophrenia is not homogeneous. If it is indeed less unitary in its symptoms, course, and underlying causal and risk factors than commonly assumed, then the overall similarity of rates may be masking differing and shifting clusters of subtypes which do not necessarily match the ICD-10/ DSM-IV fourth-digit subdivisions. This possibility is suggested by some of the findings described in the monograph. The second challenging issue concerns the highly increased risk of schizophrenia (and, possibly, mania) in first- and second-generation African-Caribbean and African immigrants. In-depth clinical and family studies are needed to test the authors' hypothesis (which has good face plausibility) that environmental pressures (and in particular, the stresses of social disadvantage) are at work in this phenomenon. In conclusion, this monograph is an excellent overview of the ideas and many of the findings generated by a highly productive group of researchers. It has a good change to become one of the standard references on several of the key aspects of schizophrenia.

Assen Jablensky

Abstract

The "epigenetic puzzle" that is schizophrenia forms the focus of this book, but we do not sit comfortably with the notion that this is an entity. Rather, we approach the psychoses on a broad epidemiological base, ascertaining cases over a quarter of a century. We examine admission policies, showing that patients are admitted to hospital on the grounds of their particular presentation, rather than their diagnosis. We explore differences between males and females with psychotic disorders, and show that gender is a more powerful influence than diagnosis. We investigate trends over time, and find that ethnicity is one of the major influences. We look at criminality, and show that the factors that predict criminal behaviour in individuals with psychotic illness are much the same as those which predict crime in the sane. We trace the longitudinal course of illness, putting paid to the schizophrenia/manic-depression dichotomy. The powerful message is that traditional diagnostic criteria are spurious, complacent constructs, which lull us into a false sense of security, and which should be challenged. We suggest that it is epidemiology which can place the current vogue for diagnostic conformity in its correct perspective, as well as provide data for service providers.

CHAPTER ONE

Schizophrenia: The epidemiology of a provisional category

This book takes the epidemiology of schizophrenia as its central theme, and focuses particularly on the way in which the disorder presents in a large city, namely London. This focus is timely because both the incidence and prevalence of the disorder are higher in large cities (Freeman, 1994), and the care (or lack of care) of psychotic patients in large cities such as London is giving rise to considerable public concern. Furthermore, there is increasing evidence that being born or brought up in an urban environment appears to increase the risk of schizophrenia (Lewis, David, Andréason, & Allebeck, 1992; Castle, Scott, Wessely, & Murray 1993).

Our research addresses such questions as whether the incidence of the disorder is changing, and which groups are at particular risk. But more than that, it uses epidemiological techniques to ask whether schizophrenia can be subdivided into more meaningful subgroups and why it appears different in men and women and in those with onset in early or late adult life. The justification for the study is that an understanding of the epidemiology of schizophrenia will not only help us to plan the facilities necessary for its optimum treatment but may also help us to find the causes of the disorder.

In this introduction, we will discuss four matters: first, general principles concerning variations in the incidence of disease and what we can learn from them; second, the advantages and disadvantages of case register studies; third, the validity of the concept of schizophrenia; and

1

finally, the implications of risk factor research for the epidemiological studies reported in this monograph.

VARIATIONS IN INCIDENCE OF DISEASE IN TIME, PLACE AND PERSON

The description of the variation in incidence of disease in different times, places, and groups of persons is the basic epidemiological challenge for relatively common disorders such as schizophrenia. Variation in disease incidence can provide important clues as to the role of environmental and/ or genetic factors in bringing on the disease (Khoury, Beatty, & Cohen, 1993; see Table 1.1)

Socioeconomic status. Social class variation in disease occurrence can provide evidence for differential exposure to environmental factors (Susser & Susser, 1987). Unfortunately, it may be difficult to identify what these factors actually are, due to the large overlap between the various factors that make up "social class", such as lifestyle, nutrition, employment, and place of residence. Of course, the fact that social class variation in disease occurrence points towards the role of environmental factors does not exclude the possibility that genetic factors confer a particular susceptibility to environmental factors (genotype–environment interaction), nor that genetic risk factors for disease play a role in social segregation (Eaton, 1980).

Geographic variation. Although geographic variation in gene frequencies for a variety of traits has been established (e.g. Sokal, 1988; Sokal, Harding, & Oden, 1989), in some instances of spacial variation, genetic factors are unlikely to play a direct role. For example, the best known example of spatial variation in the incidence of schizophrenia within

TABLE 1.1
Aetiological Implications Of Variation In Disease Occurrence In Different Settings

Epidemiological setting	Indicating the presence of:	
	Genetic factors	Environmental factors
Temporal variation	−	+
Spatial variation	(+)	+
Ethnic variation	+	+
Gender differences	+	+
Social class variation	−	+

countries is that associated with urban residence. It is unlikely that, within one and the same country, the genetic make-up of individuals living in urban areas is markedly different from that of those living in rural areas. Furthermore, for multifactorial disorders such as psychosis, with no simple one-to-one relationship between genotype and phenotype, the prevalence of disorder in urban areas would need to be many times higher than in rural areas, to confound, through genetic mechanisms, any relationship between disease incidence and urbanicity. A previous investigation has shown that this is unlikely to be the case (Lewis et al., 1992).

Therefore, geographic variation in the incidence of schizophrenia has often been interpreted as evidence for variation in environmental risk factors. Indeed, Kety (1980) has linked it to variation in risk factors associated with both urbanicity and social class by stating: "To the extent that perinatal injuries, malnutrition and infection may play a role in the environmental etiologies of schizophrenia, their impact would be exaggerated in the lower social classes in large cities." Since this monograph deals with the predominantly working-class population of Camberwell, we hope to be able to address some of these issues.

Migrant groups. The study of variation in incidence in migrant groups and their offspring can also shed light on the relative role of environmental and genetic factors. For example, if the disease in question is mostly genetically determined, disease frequency in migrant groups will closely resemble the frequency of disease in the country of origin. A similar pattern might, of course, be seen if a premigration, childhood environmental exposure in the country of origin, or an environmental exposure in the cultural "micro-environment" of the migrant family in the host country, is strongly associated with later development of disease. In the latter case, one would expect that successive generations of descendants of the migrants would show a progressively lower risk of illness. On the other hand, if environmental factors operating later in life exert a strong influence, the disease frequency in migrant groups may be expected to resemble more closely the disease frequency among individuals in the host country.

If the disease frequency in the migrant groups exceeds both that in the country of origin and the host country, then this may be an indication that the risk of the disorder is being increased either by specific factors associated with being a migrant in the host country, or by particular characteristics of the migrants, setting them apart from individuals in the host country (selective migration).

In practice, the results of migrant studies are often inconclusive. As already mentioned, migrants may be highly unrepresentative in relation to the source population, and migration status is often confounded by a host of factors including demographic characteristics, education, religion, health status, drug use, diet, access to health care, and influence of cultural pathoplastic factors on disease presentation. Furthermore, estimates of disease rates in the country of origin may be unreliable because of differences in availability of health care facilities and/or the quality of census information. Finally, migrant and ethnic groups often are difficult to define for the purposes of scientific research (McKenzie & Crowcroft, 1994), and even if they can be reliably delineated, it must be kept in mind that such groups are dynamic and undergoing continual change.

The issue of ethnic group and risk of schizophrenia is taken up in Chapters 8, 9, and 10 in which studies designed to overcome the above methodological difficulties are presented.

Gender differences. Gender-related variation in incidence has been demonstrated for many diseases such as lung cancer and coronary heart disease (more frequent in men), and autoimmune disorders (more frequent in women). Such differences sometimes provide straightforward information. For example, higher prevalence of smoking in men is likely to contribute significantly to the difference in lung cancer incidence in men and women, while the rising number of women smoking over the last decades provides a plausible explanation for the recent narrowing of this gender gap. Similarly, although the great majority of the genome in men and women is shared, simple recessive X-linked disorders occur more frequently in men because women are conferred relative protection by the presence of a second X chromosome. In general, however, the demonstration of a gender difference is only the initial step in trying to unravel the role of a host of possible genetic, social, environmental, hormonal, and occupational factors and their potential interactions.

The study of gender differences in schizophrenia has been very productive, but here also the interpretation of the findings is not straightforward. These issues will be discussed in detail in Chapters 4 and 5.

Temporal trends. Temporal trends in disease incidence in large populations are unlikely to be associated with changes in the frequency of contributing genes, and therefore point to changes in exposure to environmental risk factors. For example, in Western countries the rise in ischaemic heart disease following the 1940s is thought to have arisen from changes in the diet, while the change in incidence of poliomyelitis appears to be related to changes in exposure to protective factors (Barker, 1989).

It is very difficult, however, to show accurately trends in disease incidence, as the data used to measure disease incidence usually rely on health-care statistics, which are affected by changing diagnostic concepts and changing service provisions over time; thus, they cannot be relied on to reflect the true incidence of the disorder under study. One way of attempting to obtain more accurate information about possible temporal trends in schizophrenia and related disorders is to use data from a case register, with systematic ascertainment of cases.

THE ROLE OF CASE REGISTER STUDIES

There has been a considerable vogue in recent years for studies of schizophrenia at first onset (Lieberman et al., 1993; McGorry, Edwards, Mihalopoulos, Harrigan, & Jackson, 1996). Although an advance on studies of mixed populations of patients admitted to hospital at various points in the evolution of their illnesses, such first admission studies suffer two major disadvantages. First, they often concern admissions only, and as will be demonstrated in Chapter 3, a proportion of such individuals are not admitted during their first onset. Second, such studies do not generally draw their patients from a defined catchment area; therefore they are subject to biases in referral patterns and cannot be said to be representative of all first onset cases of schizophrenia. We have attempted to avoid these problems by using a mental health case register to identify a sample comprising of all cases of schizophrenia and related psychotic illnesses from the defined area of Camberwell in southeast London at the point of their first presentation to the psychiatric services.

Because of the various "filters" operating between the decision to seek help for mental health problems and help from specialised services (Goldberg & Huxley, 1980), only a minority of all patients with mental health disorders in a geographical area will ever be registered by a mental health case register. Most individuals deciding to seek help for "minor" mental health problems will be treated by their general practitioner. Therefore, treated incidence as measured by case register contacts will not be an accurate reflection of the total morbidity. However, disorders such as schizophrenia will result in contact with mental health services in the great majority of cases (Bamrah, Freeman, & Goldberg, 1991; Cooper et al., 1987), and the treated incidence will be more an approximation of the true incidence, especially if both community and in-patient contacts are registered (Goldacre, Shiwatch, & Yeates, 1994).

In calculating treated incidence of a disorder, diagnosis at first admission may be used, but diagnostic change can occur. It has been estimated, for example, that the incidence using first admission diagnosis is only half the incidence using diagnosis of schizophrenia ever recorded in the patient's career (Goldacre et al., 1994). Bias may occur if clinicians are differentially reluctant to apply a first diagnosis of schizophrenia with some groups, for example certain ethnic groups. This issue will be further examined in Chapters 8 and 9.

The strength of a case register lies in its epidemiological properties: (1) it covers a well-circumscribed geographical area with a well-defined population at risk; (2) it systematically registers all cases within that area who are referred for mental health treatment; (3) it registers the same data for all individuals in a standardised way. The drawbacks are that (1) data such as diagnosis and details on previous treatment are gathered in a clinical setting, which limits their reliability; (2) pathways to mental health care may differ as a function of diagnosis and other important characteristics; (3) it can only collect a minimum number of relevant variables at the expense of information on possible confounders.

The first drawback can be overcome, by including systematic checks using another source of information, such as case records (see Chapter 2). However, the second drawback cannot usually be overcome in a simple way, as pathways into care can only be established through detailed studies. Similarly, it may be difficult to obtain information on possible confounders. Case register data should therefore be used to address issues that are not entirely dependent on pathways into care and not likely to be confounded by third variables about which no information is available. Having said this, studies suggest that, in a country like England, most patients with schizophrenia do make contact with the psychiatric services in the early stages of their illness (e.g. Cooper et al., 1972).

THE VALIDITY OF THE CONCEPT OF SCHIZOPHRENIA

Any researcher carrying out a study such as ours is immediately confronted by the questions of diagnosis and definition of schizophrenia. The answers to these questions are far from simple. From the late 1960s onwards, psychiatrists spent much effort on improving the reliability of psychiatric diagnosis in general, and that for schizophrenia in particular (American Psychiatric Association, 1994; Cooper et al., 1972: Spitzer, Endicott, & Robins, 1978; Wing, Cooper & Sartorius, 1974). The result has been the development of a series of operational definitions of schizophrenia which have acceptable diagnostic reliability but, as will be seen throughout this monograph, considerable doubt as to which should be adopted. The basic problem is that we do not know whether the concept of schizophrenia has any validity, and even if it has, which operational definition best reflects that validity (Brockington, Kendell, & Leff, 1978; Crow, 1985; Murray, Lewis, & Reveley, 1985).

Part of this controversy centres on the relative merits of a narrow definition (e.g. DSM-IV; APA, 1994) or a broad definition (e.g. as in the

PSE/CATEGO system; Wing et al., 1974). This in turn arises from uncertainty concerning the boundaries of the condition, and in particular over whether differences between schizophrenia and manic-depressive psychosis are genuinely qualitative (different entities) and not merely quantitative (different values of the same entity). In their clinical practice, psychiatrists continue to use the terms schizophrenia and manic-depressive psychosis to refer to two categorically different concepts, but is the distinction into two separate categories valid?

How does one assess validity? In an ideal world, psychiatric disorders would be classified according to their different aetiologies, and validity would stem from a knowledge of aetiology. In the case of the so-called functional psychoses, we do not have definitive knowledge of aetiology but we have made some progress in establishing risk factors for the disorders; the best established of these are familial risk, cerebral ventricle size, early developmental impairment, and adverse life events. Are these risk factors specific for one particular condition, or do they operate across the psychoses?

RISK FACTORS FOR SCHIZOPHRENIA

Familial morbid risk

The existence of a genetic contribution to both schizophrenia and to manic depression is well established (Bertelson, Harvald, & Hauge, 1977; Gottesman & Shields, 1982). However, much research has shown that there is considerable overlap in familial risk between schizophrenia and affective psychosis (see review by Taylor, 1992). The Iowa 500 study found that the risks for schizophrenia in the first-degree relatives of schizophrenic, manic, and control probands were 5.5%, 3.2%, and 0.6% respectively (Tsuang, Winokur, & Crowe, 1980). Gershon and colleagues (1988) reported that the morbid risks for bipolar and unipolar disorder in the first-degree relatives of schizophrenic patients were two to three times greater than those of the relatives of non-psychiatric controls (bipolar: 2.2% vs. 0.8%; unipolar: 14.7% vs. 6.7%). Scharfetter and Nüsperli (1980) showed that the risk of bipolar disorder in the relatives of probands with catatonic schizophrenia was well above reported population figures (4.1%).

Although a number of other large and carefully conducted studies failed to show such overlap in terms of morbid risks of affective and schizophrenic psychoses in the first-degree relatives of schizophrenic and affective probands respectively (Baron, Gruen, Asnis, & Kane, 1982; Baron, Gruen, Kane, & Asnis, 1985; Coryell & Zimerman, 1988; Gershon et al., 1975), the above findings cannot be reasoned away, and no study to date has shown that schizoaffective disorder breeds true, especially schizodepressive disorder. One explanation for the discrepant findings may lie in the presence or absence of psychosis in affectively ill probands. For example, although Kendler and colleagues initially (1985) failed to find evidence for an excess of schizophrenia in the relatives of manic-depressive probands, the results changed dramatically when analyses focused on the first-degree relatives of probands with psychotic affective disorder (Kendler, Gruenberg, & Tsuang, 1986); there was an excess risk of schizophrenia in these relatives (4.3%), which even surpassed the risk for schizophrenia in the relatives of schizophrenia probands (3.7%).

Similar findings were reported in the Roscommon family study (Kendler et al., 1993), which was one of the very few such studies to use an epidemiologic approach to proband sampling. The risk for schizophrenia as determined by life-table analyses was significantly higher in the relatives of probands with schizoaffective disorder (6.7%), other non-affective psychosis (5.1%), and psychotic affective illness (2.8%), compared to the morbid risk in relatives in control probands (0.5%). These authors concluded "that the familial liability to schizophrenia is, at least in part, a liability to develop psychosis." Two recent, carefully conducted studies have also shown that the risk of schizophrenia is significantly elevated in the relatives of probands with severe bipolar disorder (Sham et al., 1994b; Vallès et al., 1996).

Thus, the evidence suggests that, rather than genetic predisposition being specific for schizophrenia, there is a continuum of genetic liability not only for the emergence of schizophrenia but of psychotic illness in general.

Cerebral ventricle dimensions

It is widely accepted that the size of the lateral cerebral ventricle is on average larger in schizophrenia patients than in well controls (Woodruff & Murray, 1994). However, there is considerable overlap in the distributions of ventricular size in schizophrenic and normal populations. Furthermore, Jones and colleagues (1994b) demonstrated a linear trend in the association between lateral ventricle size and schizophrenia, which indicates that risk is not confined to a subgroup with very large ventricles, but rather that ventricular enlargement is best conceived as a continuous risk factor: the larger the ventricles, the greater the risk of schizophrenia.

Furthermore, the association does not appear to be specific to schizophrenia but appears less strong in the affective psychoses (Andreasen, Swayze, Flaum, Alliger, & Cohen, 1990; Harvey, Persaud, Ron, Barker, & Murray, 1994; Jones et al., 1994b). An early study by Weinberger and colleagues (1982) suggests that there is a gradient of risk, the strongest risk of enlarged ventricles being associated with persistent schizophrenia (mean VBR = 6.0), declining through schizophreniform disorder (VBR = 5.3) to affective disorder (VBR = 3.8), and control values (VBR = 2.9). A recent careful meta-analysis by Elkis, Friedman, Wise, & Meltzer (1995) shows that both cerebral ventricle size and sulcal prominence are risk factors for both affective disorder and schizophrenia, but with a larger effect size in the latter.

Thus, one cannot argue convincingly that the subtle structural abnormalities which are found in the brains of people with schizophrenia are specific for that condition. Once again, the risk appears to be in part shared by patients with another psychotic condition, namely affective psychosis.

Early developmental impairment

Early developmental attenuation has been shown to be a risk factor for later schizophrenia (Jones, Rodgers, Murray, & Marmot, 1994a). Once again, the specificity of this finding remains in doubt, as evidence has emerged suggesting that individuals with affective disorder and non-schizophrenic psychosis show neurological abnormalities and subtle differences in social and cognitive development, similar to those found in patients with schizophrenia, although less marked (Rodgers, 1990; Done, Sacker, & Crow, 1994; Van Os et al., 1997a). For example, in a study of a population-based sample of 387 patients with non-depressive functional psychoses, we examined proxy measures of developmental deviance, such as poor academic achievement, prepsychotic unemployment, and single marital status (Van Os et al., 1996c). Compared to individuals with mania, patients with chronic schizophrenia had a three to six times increased risk of reported prepsychotic deficits. For patients with schizomania and acute schizophrenia, the risk was 1.5–3 times greater than for manic patients. These findings suggest that the degree of developmental deficit varies as a function both of disorder and of its persistence: manic patients have the lowest risk of prepsychotic deficits and the best outcome; those with chronic schizophrenia a high risk of both prepsychotic deviance and poor outcome; and those with schizomania and acute schizophrenia somewhere in between.

Life events

In spite of the many methodological difficulties in measuring life events, a consensus exists that adverse life events precede affective psychosis more frequently than one would expect. However, the results of seven studies reviewed by Bebbington et al. (1993) also suggested an excess of stressful life events in the three weeks before onset of schizophrenic illness. Recent support for this association between life events and illness onset has come from three studies that introduced important methodological improvements such as prospective designs, inclusion of appropriate controls, and rating of severity and degree of threat of the life event (Bebbington et al., 1993; Malla, Cortese, Shaw, & Ginsberg, 1990; Ventura, Neuchterlein, Lukoff, & Hardisty, 1989).

Thus, the association between life events and illness onset is not specific to any particular diagnostic category within the functional psychoses. Nevertheless, there is some evidence that the effect sizes are greater in affective illnesses than in schizophrenia. For example, Paykel (1978) calculated the relative risk to express the magnitude of the association between life events and onset of disorder. He found that the risk of developing depression increased sixfold in the six months after experiencing markedly threatening life events. However, the comparable increase in risk for schizophrenia was two- to fourfold. In our own recent study (Bebbington et al., 1993), we found that the risk of developing psychotic depression was increased sevenfold, compared to a fivefold increase for schizophrenia. Similar results were recently reported by Dohrenwend and colleagues (1995).

THE IMPLICATIONS FOR OUR STUDIES

We conclude from the last two sections on validity and risk factors that, first, the orthodox psychiatric belief that schizophrenia and manic-depressive psychosis are discrete entities is unproven; and, second, there is little evidence that any risk factor is specific to any diagnostic category within the functional psychoses. However, the magnitude of these risk factors for psychotic illness appears to vary as a function of baseline psychopathology, such that the associations between onset of psychosis and familial morbid risk of schizophrenia, cerebral ventricle size, and premorbid adjustment are most evident at the schizophrenic end of the spectrum, and those for life events and for familial morbid risk of affective disorder are more evident at the affective end.

Such findings are suggestive of a psychopathological continuum with discrete effects working preferentially, though not exclusively, at particular ends of the continuum. There appears to be a gradient in terms of the magnitude of the effect of risk factors, along the continuum, rather than qualitative distinctions between categories. The supposition of discrete effects operating in varying strength at different ends of a psychopathological continuum is a conceptually coherent starting point for further investigation, and has some advantages over the search for separate risk factors for onset of diagnostic constructs of uncertain validity.

Should we, therefore, abandon the concept of schizophrenia in our studies, and instead examine the epidemiology of psychosis as a whole? Kendell and Zealley (1993) point out that in psychiatry, there is no absolute preference for classifications based on differences by kind or by degree, and that the choice of classification depends on the issue which one wants to address. We may see the same two entities as alike on certain occasions, and as unlike on other occasions, depending upon our purposes. If the purpose is better understanding of the determinants of psychosis, then it seems logical to adhere to the view that there are differences by degree, and not by kind between different diagnostic categories.

However, for epidemiological research it is convenient to work with "cases" of a disorder, yielding easily interpretable measures of disease frequency and risk factor effect sizes. We shall therefore report findings later in this book concerning schizophrenia but it is important to keep in mind that, in the "case" of schizophrenia, this can be no more than a working hypothesis at one end of the psychosis continuum.

CONCLUSION

In conclusion, the research we report in this book examines the epidemiology of schizophrenia and related illnesses in Inner London. We adopt the classic epidemiological stance in seeking to describe the incidence of the disorders, and in time trends in incidence, in relation to factors such as age, gender, social class, and ethnicity. Nevertheless, we do so in the knowledge that schizophrenia may be no more than a provisional category, and therefore adopt a broad definition of cases of psychosis to be included. We examine risk factors such as family history or developmental impairment for the conditions as a whole in various subpopulations of cases: the young/the old, males/females, white/African-Caribbean. Most importantly, we use a case register to identify cases and to ensure that the population of first onset patients that we examine is a representative one.

CHAPTER TWO

Methods for the 1965–1984 study

This book describes the epidemiology of schizophrenia and related disorders in Camberwell, in southeast London. It mainly utilises data collected over the period 1965–1984 through the Camberwell Cumulative Psychiatric Case Register (Wing & Hailey, 1972). However, for the analyses on trends in the incidence of schizophrenia, and the influence of ethnicity on such trends, data up to 1992 were incorporated. This enabled us to take advantage of data from the 1991 national census, the first to include an item on perceived ethnicity, allowing a more accurate estimation of the denominator in these analyses. Finally, we take forward a number of issues raised by the Camberwell Register data, in describing findings from a prospective series of Camberwell patients ascertained as part of a separate study, the Camberwell Collaborative Psychosis Study. The patients included in that sample represent a subgroup of Camberwell patients with psychotic disorders, who made contact with the psychiatric services over the years 1986 to 1989; hence, the sampling frame is the same as that from which the participants described in the main part of this book, were drawn.

The methodology of the trends/ethnicity and Camberwell Collaborative Psychosis Study are described in Chapters 10 and 11. Here we confine ourselves to a description of the 1965–1984 sample.

To place our findings in context, we first provide a brief description of the demography of the population living in the Camberwell catchment area over the period of study. An overall outline of the methodology of the study then follows. More specific methodological issues are addressed in the relevant chapters.

THE CAMBERWELL CATCHMENT AREA

The Camberwell catchment area is a deprived inner-city area in southeast London, England, which is geographically congruent with the southern portion of the London borough of Southwark. The demography of the area's population changed considerably over the 20-year period (1965–1984) of operation of the Camberwell Register. Population numbers for the Camberwell catchment area, by sex and age, for each year of the study were derived from small area statistics from the 1961, 1971, and 1981 censuses (100% samples), with interpolations for intermediate years.

The total population declined from 171,000 in 1965 to 118,000 in 1981. Overall, however, there has been remarkably little change in the age structure of the population in the years under study. In 1965, 38% of males and 35% of females were under 25, and 66% of males and 61% of females under 45. The comparable figures for 1981 were 37% of males and 35% of females under 25, and 65% of males and 61% of females under 45. The male:female ratio also remained stable over the years (48% male in both 1965 and 1981). National figures for England and Wales are very similar; for example, the 1981 census shows that 38% of males and 34% of females were under the age of 25, and 65% and 60%, respectively, under the age of 45.

Camberwell rates highly on deprivation indices based on factors such as housing tenure and socioeconomic status (see Balarajan, Yuen, & Machin, 1992), and consequently is above average in terms of measures of such deprivation, the so-called Jarman indices. An overrepresentation of individuals in lower socioeconomic groupings has been a longstanding characteristic of the area. Table 2.1 shows socioeconomic groupings for the area in the 1961, 1971, and 1981 censuses. The proportion of individuals in social classes IV and V increased, albeit slightly, over the study period. In contrast, figures for England as a whole show that the proportion of individuals in social classes IV and V declined modestly over this period (see Table 2.1).

Although the general population of Camberwell decreased over the decades following the 1961 census, there was a marked growth in the proportion of migrant groups in the population. In particular, there has been an influx into the area of persons born in the Caribbean, the proportion in the general population rising from 2.5% in the 1961 census to 6.6% in the 1981 census. As these individuals came to the UK in their early adulthood, and have subsequently produced children, African-

TABLE 2.1

Socioeconomic Groupings For Camberwell Catchment Area And England As A Whole, 1961, 1971 And 1981 Censuses

Social class	1961 England	1966 Southwark Borough*	1971		1981	
			England	Camberwell	England	Camberwell
I	3.8	2.3	5.1	6.2	5.9	5.8
II	15.2	6.2	18.2	6.7	23.0	12.4
III—Non-manual		18.6	12.3	21.1	12.0	20.0
III—Manual	51.3	39.3	38.2	36.1	36.1	33.2
IV	20.7	17.8	17.9	15.8	16.8	18.6
V	9.0	15.8	8.3	11.5	6.2	10.0

* The borough into which Camberwell catchment area falls; 1961 small area statistics for SE groupings not available from OPCS.

Caribbean people in Camberwell are generally younger than their (UK-born) Caucasian counterparts.

Regrettably, none of the general population censuses prior to 1991 collected information specifically about ethnicity. Thus, for assessment of ethnic composition of the area over the course of the study, up to the 1991 census period, we had to rely on data on "country of origin of head of household" to provide a proxy measure of ethnic composition of the household.

Sampling frame

The case-finding strategy was to ascertain all patients with non-affective functional psychoses, from a defined catchment area, who made their first psychiatric contact over a defined period. To achieve this, use was made of the Camberwell Cumulative Psychiatric Case Register (Wing & Hailey, 1972), which provides a comprehensive list of all persons from the area of Camberwell, who had their first contact with the psychiatric services between 1965 and 1984. A list was generated from the Register of all first contacts in the following diagnostic categories: schizophrenia and related conditions (equivalent ICD-9 codes 295.0 to 259.9), including schizoaffective disorder (ICD 295.7); "paraphrenia" (ICD 297.2); and "other functional psychoses" (ICD 298.1 to 298.9). In accord with the principles set out in Chapter 1, this broad range of diagnoses was chosen to avoid preselection according to any specific set of diagnostic criteria or age at onset, and to allow for changes in diagnostic habit over time.

Diagnosis

The case-records of each patient were obtained from the appropriate hospital or clinic, and all medical, nursing, social work, and occupational therapy notes were scrutinised, as well as all correspondence and accessory information. The quality of the written notes was high, and in most cases a semistandardised case summary was also available, prepared according to the format outlined by the Institute of Psychiatry Training Committee (1973). Patients who had had contact with the psychiatric services prior to 1965 were excluded from further analysis, as were patients in whom there was an obvious organic basis to the illness.

Demographic variables

A checklist was compiled for completion on each individual; this is reproduced as Appendix 1. Specific items of importance to the analyses presented in this book are: sex, age at first psychiatric contact, date of birth, and ethnicity and country of birth of patient and parents. Ethnicity categories were Caucasian, Afro-Caribbean, Asian and "other", while "country of birth" categories were UK and Eire, West Indies (Caribbean), Asia, Africa, and "other". These data were recorded directly from the case records; checks on date of contact, date of birth, and country of origin were made from the front sheets of the case records, and the Camberwell Register itself. Checks on ethnicity ratings were made on a subset of 34 patients, using data from previous direct interview studies involving these patients; no erroneous ratings were found. Further checks on ethnicity ratings are detailed in Chapter 9.

Definitions of illness

The Operational Criteria Checklist for Psychotic Illness or OCCPI, version 2.5 (McGuffin, Farmer, & Harvey, 1991) was completed for each individual. The checklist, reproduced in full as Appendix 1c, provides a simple, reliable method of applying multiple operational diagnostic criteria in studies of psychotic illness. The precise definition of each item is given in Appendix 2. The OCCPI 2.5 checklist is allied to a computer software programme, OPCRIT, which generates diagnoses according to operational criteria. For the purposes of our studies, ICD (WHO, 1978) diagnoses were taken as akin to a Register diagnosis of "schizophrenia" (ICD-9 codes 295.0–.9), "schizoaffective disorder" (ICD 295.7), "paraphrenia" (ICD 297.2), or "other non-organic psychosis" (298.1–.9). Research Diagnostic Criteria (RDC; Spitzer et al., 1978), DSM-III and DSM-III-R (American Psychiatric Association, 1980, 1987) and Feighner (Feighner et al., 1972) diagnoses were derived using the OPCRIT computer programme. OPCRIT treats missing values as 0.

For the Camberwell Register cases (i.e. those ascertained between 1965 and 1984), DJC and SW each rated approximately half the case records. Interrater reliability was computed on a random subset of 50 case notes which were independently rated by both workers; kappa was 0.82 for RDC diagnoses and 0.76, 0.74, and 0.76 for DSM-III, DSM-III-R, and Feighner diagnoses, respectively.

Age-at-onset and premorbid variables

Age-at-onset was recorded as "the earliest age at which medical advice was sought for psychiatric reasons or at which symptoms began to cause subjective distress or impair functioning" (as in OCCPI). Interrater reliability (performed by five-year bands) for age at onset was excellent (kappa = 0.93). Information relating to marital/cohabiting status at time of contact, and to premorbid social and work adjustment, as well as the presence or absence of abnormal premorbid personality traits was also rated, in accordance with the criteria laid down in the OCCPI.

"Premorbid" refers to the period before the onset of illness, as defined above. The criteria for poor premorbid work adjustment take account of poor academic work and of poor performance as a housewife, thus reducing bias relating to early onset patients (scholars/students) or females (housewives). For the premorbid variables, interrater reliabilities (kappa) were single: 1.0; premorbid work adjustment: 0.65; premorbid social adjustment: 0.64; and personality disorder: 0.60.

CHAPTER THREE

Diagnostic issues and admission policies

For the period of operation of the Camberwell Register (i.e. 1965–1984), there were 566 patients on the Register in the appropriate categories. Case records were obtained on 517 (91%). For six of these patients the case records were of insufficient quality to allow rating, and these were counted as "missing" in further analyses. The number of patients for whom case records were missing differed over the years under study. Thus, in the 1965–1969 cohort, 19 records were missing (14% of the total potential cases in that cohort), 22 (17%) in the 1970–1974 cohort, 11 (8%) in the 1975–1980 cohort, and 3 (2%) in the 1980–1984 cohort. The greater proportion of missing notes in the first decade of the study is due to a number of these notes having been destroyed due to lack of storage space at one of the local hospitals. There is no reason to suspect that this administrative vandalism introduced any systematic bias. Specifically, there were no significant differences in the distribution of Register diagnoses, the proportion of males, or the proportion of individuals born outside the UK; also, the age structure was similar.

Of the 511 available cases, 15 had had previous psychiatric contact elsewhere, or contact before 1965. The Register specifically aimed to exclude such individuals, but the 15 discovered in the "double check", who do not contribute to the incidence rate of schizophrenia, were excluded. In a further six patients, the illness had an obvious organic basis (such as delirium tremens or neurosyphilis), and in a further four, the patients did not receive a psychiatric diagnosis at time of contact. Thus, the final sample comprised 486 valid cases. Some of the analyses presented in this book exclude a few further cases if the relevant data were missing; the exact sample size in each set of analyses is given in the appropriate chapter, and where necessary (e.g. in assessing rates), adjustments were made for missing cases.

DIAGNOSTIC CRITERIA FULFILLED

Table 3.1 shows the diagnostic breakdown according to RDC, DSM-III, DSM-III-R and Feighner criteria. As such, the distributions reflect differences in emphasis between these sets of criteria for psychotic disorders. For example, Feighner criteria for "definite" schizophrenia include an age-at-onset cut-off at 40 years, and a positive family history of schizophrenia; only 32% of cases met these criteria. DSM-III and DSM-III-R criteria both stipulate a six-month illness duration for a diagnosis of schizophrenia. This results in many patients with a shorter illness duration being relegated to the "schizophreniform psychosis" or "atypical psychosis" categories. RDC are the most liberal for schizophrenia, with no age-at-onset stipulation, and only a two-week duration requirement. Indeed, nearly two-thirds of cases met RDC criteria for schizophrenia.

DSM-III does not allow a diagnosis of schizophrenia if the illness first manifested after the age of 44 years, whilst DSM-III-R removed this stipulation. Many later onset cases would, under DSM-III rules, be subsumed under the "atypical psychosis" category; indeed, over a third of cases were in this group in DSM-III. DSM-III-R not only allowed a diagnosis of schizophrenia in patients with a late onset of illness, but also introduced the "delusional disorder" category, which is similar to the Kraepelinian concept of paranoia (see Munro, 1988). Over 10% of cases were labelled "delusional disorder" under DSM-III-R rules. A more detailed discussion of early- and late-onset cases is given in Chapter 6.

There are also considerable differences in the proportion of males and females fulfilling various sets of diagnostic criteria for schizophrenia. These gender differences are presented in Chapters 4 and 5.

The very few cases assigned to the affective spectrum is due to the selection of cases to include only "non-affective" psychoses. The fact that around 10% of cases fulfilled DSM-III and DSM-III-R criteria for "schizoaffective disorder" reflects the uncertain nosological status of such cases; this is discussed further in Chapter 5. The "no diagnosis" categories are recorded because the OCCPI 2.5 system uses only psychotic diagnostic categories, and the sets of criteria used, do not allocate every case to a diagnostic category. The absence of alcohol and drug-related diagnoses reflects the fact that they are coded separately on the Camberwell Register, and that OPCRIT does not code for them.

TABLE 3.1

Number (Percentage) Of Patients Fulfilling Various Criteria For Functional Psychotic Illness

RDC	*Major depression* 31 (6.3%)	*Mania/ bipolar* 14 (2.8%)	*Schizoaffective mania* 16 (3.3%)	*Schizoaffective depression* 11 (2.3%)	*"Broad" schizophrenia* 50 (10.3%)	*"Narrow" schizophrenia* 271 (55.8%)	*"Other"/no diagnosis* 93 (4.1%)
DSM-III	*Major depression* 8 (1.6%)	*Bipolar* 1 (0.2%)	*Schizoaffective* 44 (9.1%)	*Atypical psychosis* 181 (37.2%)	*Schizophreniform* 74 (15.2%)	*Schizophrenia* 158 (32.6%)	*"Other"/no diagnosis* 20 (4.1%)
DSM-III-R	*Major depression* 10 (2.0%)	*Bipolar* 1 (0.2%)	*Schizoaffective* 59 (12.1%)	*Atypical psychosis* 94 (19.3%)	*Schizophreniform* 53 (10.9%)	*Schizophrenia* 196 (40.4%)	*Delusional disorder* 51 (10.6%) *"Other"/no diagnosis* 22 (4.5%)
Feighner					*Probable schizophrenia* 87 (17.9%)	*Definite schizophrenia* 157 (32.3%)	*"Other"/no diagnosis*

ADMISSION POLICIES

One of the crucial advantages of the current study over many of those in the literature is that the sample under consideration consisted of consecutive first contacts rather than relying on admission data. In order to assess the biases which might have arisen had only patients admitted to hospital been considered, the demographic and diagnostic differences between those patients admitted at first psychiatric contact, and those not admitted, were analysed. These analyses are based on the entire sample of 486 valid cases (i.e. ICD-9 codes 295, 297.2, 298). Unless otherwise specified, results are presented as risk ratios (RR) with 95% confidence intervals (95% CI). A fuller exposition can be found in Castle, Sham, Wessely, and Murray (1994).

Trends over time and demographic variables

Trends in admission practices over time were assessed by determining the proportion of patients admitted to hospital at first psychiatric contact by five-year date bands. The percentages of admitted patients were 79, 82, 77, and 74% for the 1965–1969, 1970–1974, 1975–1979, and 1980–1984 date bands, respectively (M–H test for trend chi-square = 1.77; 1df; P = .18).

Of patients born in the UK/Eire, 80% were admitted at first contact, compared with 75% of those born in the West Indies and 60% of those born in Asia; the differences were not significant, probably because of the small number of Asian born. Comparison of ethnic Caucasians with ethnic African-Caribbeans did not reveal any significant difference in proportion admitted (79% and 78% respectively). The following factors also failed to predict admission to hospital: sex (males = 77%, females = 79%; RR = 1.13; 95% CI = 0.74–1.74); married/cohabiting status (married/cohabiting = 79%; single = 78%; RR = 0.92; 95% CI = 0.59–1.43); and being unemployed (unemployed = 78%; employed = 79%; RR = 0.95; 95% CI = 0.60–1.48).

The fact that gender, age-at-onset, and marital and employment status did not act as predictors of admission is unexpected. Early-onset male schizophrenia patients tend to have a severe disorder (see Chapters 4 and 5) and one might have expected them more likely to be admitted. Furthermore, marriage is purported to have a "protective" effect in schizophrenia, while employment would suggest a relatively high level of functioning in the community. Indeed, these findings are at odds with the experience of groups who have specifically focused on managing acutely ill psychiatric patients outside hospitals. For example, a home-based team in Birmingham (Dean & Gadd, 1990) found that being single and living alone both predicted admission, while being young predicted admission for male (but not female) patients.

Substance use

Patients with a history of problem drinking or alcohol dependence were less likely to be admitted than those without such a history (71% vs. 81%), but the difference was not statistically significant (RR = 0.59; 95% CI = 0.33–1.08). A similar but significant trend was seen for patients with a history of cannabis abuse (65% vs. 81%; RR = 0.44; 95% CI = 0.23–0.85).

It is difficult to interpret these findings in that patients with substance abuse often have florid psychoses and show behavioural disturbance; these parameters actually predicted admission, as is detailed below, and this is seemingly at odds with the data on substance use. It may be that psychiatrists tend to be wary about admitting patients with possible drug-induced psychoses.

Criminality and violence

A history of juvenile delinquency or adult criminality was slightly less common in patients admitted to hospital; again, differences were not significant. However, if police were involved in bringing the patient to hospital, there was a 93% chance of admission, compared to 79% if there was no such history (RR = 3.61; 95% CI = 1.27–10.26). Violence to others was likely to result in admission (91% vs. 78%; RR = 2.74; 95% CI = 1.22–6.20), while all patients with a history of violence to self were admitted to hospital vs 80% of those with no such history (RR = 0.79; 95% CI = 0.76–0.84).

Thus, whilst past forensic history had no significant influence on admission, police involvement in the process of referral was a predictor of admission, as was violence to others. This indicates that it is current behaviour that has the strongest influence on admission policy.

Clinical characteristics

Phenomenological variables, as defined in OCCPI 2.5, were compared in patients admitted to hospital with those not admitted. Those variables considered are shown in Table 3.2. The characteristics associated with admission included persecutory and grandiose delusions, and any form of hallucination. More classically "schizophrenic" phenomena, such as passivity and thought insertion and withdrawal, were no more common in patients admitted to hospital than in those not admitted; this was not merely an artifact due to the relatively low frequency of such phenomena, as evidenced by the percentage distributions shown in Table 3.2. Of interest is that patients who lacked insight into their condition were more likely to be admitted.

TABLE 3.2
Phenomenological Variables Of Patients Admitted

Variable	No. with symptom	% with admitted	% without admitted	Risk ratio; 95% CI
Lack of insight	215	82	48	4.94; 2.69–9.06
Catatonia	27	89	78	2.23; 0.65–7.57
Positive formal thought disorder	107	83	77	1.45; 0.82–2.54
Negative formal thought disorder	41	88	79	2.06; 0.78–5.39
Blunting of affect	10	80	79	1.08; 0.22–5.21
Persecutory delusions	368	82	68	2.05; 1.27–3.33
Systematised delusions	139	79	79	1.03; 0.63–1.67
Grandiose delusions	102	87	77	2.10; 1.12–3.95
Delusions of reference	297	88	76	1.23; 0.79–1.91
Bizarre delusions	109	82	78	1.27; 0.74–2.19
Widespread delusions	235	83	75	1.59; 1.02–2.49
Passivity phenomena	123	81	78	1.25; 0.74–2.09
Delusional perception	17	65	79	0.48; 0.17–1.34
Other primary delusions	52	71	80	0.63; 0.33–1.20
Persecutory hallucinations	279	86	68	3.02; 1.92–4.76
Thought insertion	61	72	80	0.66; 0.36–1.22
Thought withdrawal	33	85	78	1.56; 0.59–4.16
Thought broadcast	45	76	79	0.82; 0.40–1.69
Thought echo	10	70	79	0.62; 0.16–2.47
3rd person hallucinations	157	84	76	1.66; 1.01–2.75
Running commentary	81	88	77	2.10; 1.04–4.24

Behavioural items such as bizarre behaviour (86% in those admitted to hospital vs. 73% in those not admitted; RR = 2.18; 95% CI = 1.36–3.47) and reckless activity (95% vs. 77%; RR = 6.09; 95% CI = 1.45–25.63) also predicted admission. Manic symptoms of elevated mood (90% vs. 77%; RR = 2.49; 95% CI = 0.86–7.19) or irritable mood (89% vs. 77%; RR = 2.51; 95% CI = 1.04–6.04) also tended to be associated with admission.

These findings suggest that florid persecutory ideation and behavioural disturbance were more likely to influence admission practice than textbook "typically schizophrenic" symptoms. This is underlined by the fact that patients with a diagnosis of schizoaffective disorder or DSM-III–R schizophreniform psychosis were most likely to be admitted (90% of the former and 89% of latter being admitted at first contact, compared with 83% of patients with "schizophrenia").

Patients with schizoaffective disorder and schizophreniform psychosis tend to have florid symptomatology and often exhibit disruptive behaviour. In contrast, fewer than two-thirds of patients with DSM-III–R delusional disorder were admitted. Typically, patients with this disorder exhibit non-bizarre delusions without prominent hallucinations, and are often not behaviourally disturbed (APA, 1987).

DISCUSSION

Around 20% of patients with a non-affective psychosis were not admitted on first contact with the psychiatric services. This figure is remarkably similar to that reported by Shepherd, Watt & Falloon (1989) that 20% of schizophrenia patients being admitted to hospital for the first time had had a previous episode of illness for which they had not been admitted. Perhaps surprisingly, the proportion of admitted patients in the current study did not change much over the years. Trends towards community psychiatric care (Prince & Phelan, 1990), as well as the wider use of depot neuroleptic medication (Graham, 1990), might have been expected to lead to a reduction in the number of patients requiring admission. Our findings probably reflect a relatively stable service provision, and lend credence to the assessment of trends in incidence detailed in Chapter 8.

The finding of floridly behaviourally disturbed violent patients who are most likely to admitted to hospital at first contact underlines the bias which could arise in samples of hospitalised samples.

CHAPTER FOUR

The effect of gender on age at onset of psychosis

Gender differences in the functional psychoses form the focus of the following two chapters. This chapter deals with gender differences in mean age at onset of illness, investigates potential confounders of such differences, and explores age at onset distribution curves for men and women. The following chapter takes forward the findings in the form of a latent class analysis.

SEX DIFFERENCES IN AGE AT ONSET IN SCHIZOPHRENIA

It has been widely reported that men have a mean onset of schizophrenia earlier than women (reviewed by Angermeyer, Goldstein, & Kuhn, 1988; Lewine, 1988). Most studies report the extent of the difference to be around five years (see Lewine, 1988). Gender differences in onset are not an artifact due to definition of illness, being found even if stringent DSM-III (APA, 1980) criteria are employed (Loranger, 1984; Shimizu et al., 1988). There is also consistency across cultures, in that an analysis of data from 11 centres of the WHO determinants of outcome study (Hambrecht, Maurer, Hafner, & Sartorius, 1992) found that females had a later onset than males in all centres.

Explanations of the age at onset difference in terms of confounding factors have generally been refuted. For example, differences in help-seeking behaviour between males and females with schizophrenia, or by their families, cannot explain away the findings; however "onset" is defined (first treatment, first hospitalisation, first symptoms), the sex differences in age at onset are robust (Hafner, Behrens, De Vry, & Gattaz, 1991; Loranger, 1984; Riecher et al., 1989). Faroane, Chen, Goldstein, and Tsuang (1994), using the Iowa 500 sample, investigated the possible confounding effects of longevity in women in the general population, and the differential proneness of males with schizophrenia to early death. Even controlling for the age composition of the population of origin and allowing for the differential mortality, age at onset was later in females than males with schizophrenia. One psychosocial factor which remains a potential confounding variable in the differential age at onset in schizophrenia is marital status. Thus, Hafner and colleagues (1989), using a case register sample, found that, if only single men and women with schizophrenia were considered, the age at onset differential between the sexes disappeared. More recently, Jablensky and Cole (1997), using data from the WHO determinants of outcome study, also suggested that marital status confounds the gender difference in age at onset. These authors examined 778 men and 653 women in 10 countries to estimate the unconfounded contributions of gender, family history, premorbid personality, and marital status on age at onset. They report strong main effects for marital status and premorbid personality, a weak effect for family history, and no effect for gender. These findings underline the potential importance of psychosocial factors in explaining gender differences in schizophrenia.

A further relatively underexplored fact about gender differences in onset of schizophrenia, and one often disguised in studies which report only mean differences, is that the age at onset distribution curves for men and women differ markedly from each other. For example, in a study of 392 consecutive first admissions with a diagnosis of schizophrenia or paranoid disorder from a defined catchment area, Hafner and colleagues (1991) found that males showed a single marked peak in the early 20s, while for females there was a "second peak" of onset in the 45–54 year age group. This finding was echoed in the distribution of pooled data from the WHO determinants of outcome study (Hambrecht et al., 1992).

Even these aforementioned studies, however, sampled only patients with an onset of illness below their mid-50s. Despite the plethora of epidemiological investigations in schizophrenia, late-onset illness has all too often been ignored. The reasons (until recently) for this lack of interest in schizophrenia with its first manifestation in late life lie, in part at least, in the tacit acceptance (expressly in the US, and embodied in DSM-III criteria for schizophrenia), that schizophrenia cannot manifest for the first time after 44 years of age (APA, 1980). The European tradition has been somewhat different, and ICD-9 (WHO, 1978) does not have an age at onset stipulation for schizophrenia; furthermore, paraphrenia, akin to Roth's (1955) concept of "late paraphrenia" as a paranoid delusional illness with onset usually after the age of 60, was recognised in ICD-9, though it has been dropped from ICD-10 (WHO, 1993).

Gender differences in late-onset schizophrenia have been widely reported, with a female excess found in almost all studies of late onset schizophrenia which have included both sexes. The female:male ratio in the over-40s ranges from 5:3 (Bland, 1977) to 1.9:1 (Bleuler, 1943); in very late-onset cases (onset > 60 years), the female preponderance is even more marked, ranging from 3:1 (Roth, 1955) to 45:2 (Herbert & Jacobsen, 1967).

The analyses presented in this chapter aim to exploit the sampling frame afforded by the Camberwell Register. Thus, using a catchment area sample not biased by admission, and which included all non-affective psychotic patients without any exclusion of patients with a late onset of illness, we were able to: (1) assess the sex difference in mean age at onset; (2) report the full onset curves for men and women across all ages; (3) investigate the effect of diagnostic stringency on the sex-distribution curves; and (4) ascertain the influence of premorbid and psychosocial factors on age at onset in men and women.

THE CURRENT STUDY

Incidence

Rates of schizophrenia by gender were determined by five-year date bands across the study period 1965–1984, using data supplied by the Office for Population Censuses and Surveys (OPCS). Data from the 1961, 1971 and 1981 censuses (100% samples) were used, with appropriate interpolations for the intermediate years. The male:female ratio of the general population of Camberwell was fairly uniform throughout the period under study, showing a slight female preponderance. The male:female rate ratios were thus much the same over the 20 years, and results are shown for the whole group. For all diagnoses, there were 248 males (51%) and 238 females (49%).

Figure 4.1 shows the age at onset distribution for all non-affective non-organic psychotic patients, by gender. Mean age at onset was 31.2 years (SD 14.9) for males and 41.1 years (SD 20.7) for females ($t = -6.02$; 475 df; $P < .0001$). Males exceeded females in those patients with an onset before the age of 36 years, whereas after that age a female preponderance was seen.

The age-at-onset differential between the sexes was not fully accounted for by those schizophrenia spectrum disorders included in the whole sample, as the differential was found even when analyses were restricted to patients fulfilling operationalised criteria for schizophrenia. Indeed, this

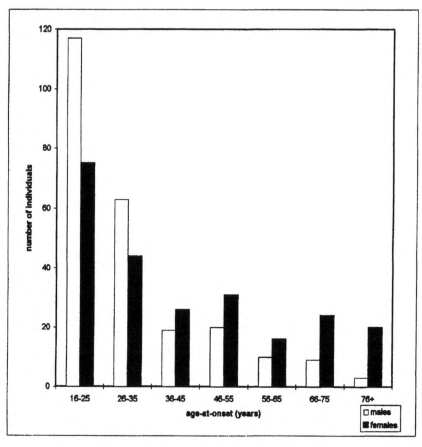

FIG. 4.1.   Age-at-onset distribution for all non-affective non-organic psychotic patients, by gender.

was true even for those men and women fulfilling restrictive DSM-III (APA, 1980) criteria for schizophrenia, which has an age at onset cut off at 45 years; thus, mean onset for males with DSM-III schizophrenia ($n = 108$) was 24.8 years (SD 6.6), and for females ($n = 50$) 27.5 years (SD 8.5), a statistically significant difference ($t = -2.2$; 156 df; $P < .03$).

The effect of marital status and other psychosocial variables

Of the 477 patients included in this set of analyses, 270 (57%) were single at time of onset of illness; of these, 161 (60%) were male. In contrast, of the married/cohabiting patients, only 38% were male.

For the single patients, males had a mean age at onset of 26.0 years (*SD* 11.3), and females 35.1 years (*SD* 20.2), a highly significant difference ($t = -4.72$; 268 *df*; $P < .0001$). However, when only married/cohabiting patients were considered, the age at onset differential for men and women all but disappeared (males 42.1 years (*SD* 16.0); females 46.5 years (*SD* 19.7); $t = -1.66$; 201 *df*; $P = .10$).

We proceeded to investigate other "premorbid" psychosocial parameters in terms of their influence on the gender difference in age at onset. Patients with a poor premorbid employment history had an earlier onset of illness than those without such a history (27.7 years (*SD* 12.0) vs. 41.5 years (*SD* 20.2); $t = 8.43$; 469 *df*; $P < .0001$). A similar trend was found for those individuals with poor premorbid social adjustment (30.2 years (*SD* 15.6) vs. 39.4 years (*SD* 19.4; $t = 5.33$; 470 *df*; $P < .0001$). However, adjustment for poor premorbid occupational and social adjustment did not affect the gender difference in age at onset, as is shown in Table 4.1a and b.

We also considered whether, as had been reported in a number of studies (e.g. Sham et al., 1994a,b), patients with a family history of schizophrenia had an earlier onset of illness than those without such a history. In fact, patients with a positive family history did have an earlier mean onset of illness (mean 30.3 years (*SD* 15.8) compared with 36.4 years (*SD* 19.1)), but this difference narrowly missed statistical significance at the 5% level ($t = 1.85$; 449 *df*; $P = .06$).

Sex and premorbid parameters in early- and late-onset patients

To explore further the influence of premorbid functioning on age at onset in the current sample, and particularly to assess whether gender confounded any of the associations, we dichotomised the sample by the mean (i.e. 36 years), for use as the dependent variable.

Patients with an onset of illness before the age of 36 ("early onset": $n = 299$) were, in comparison with those with an onset over 35 years ("late onset": $n = 178$), more likely to be single (71% vs. 34%; RR = 0.21; 95% CI = 0.14–0.32) and to have exhibited poor premorbid social adjustment (47% vs. 19%; RR = 0.27; 95% CI = 0.17–0.42). They were also more likely to have a poor work record premorbidly (53% vs. 19%; RR = 0.21; 95% CI = 0.13–0.32), and to exhibit personality dysfunction (23% vs. 7%; RR = 0.26; 95% CI = 0.14–0.48).

As we were particularly interested in the possible confounding and interaction effects of gender on these associations, we examined men and women separately in terms of these same parameters. Thus, in the total sample, males were more likely to be single (68% vs. 46%; RR = 0.41;

TABLE 4.1a
Gender Difference In Age At Onset, By Premorbid Work Adjustment

Premorbid work adjustment	Mean (SD) age at onset (yrs)		t-Value	df	P-Value
	males	females			
Good	36.7 (17.2)	45.3 (21.6)	−3.60	280	.000
Poor	24.5 (7.6)	32.3 (15.2)	−4.64	187	.000

TABLE 4.1b
Gender Difference In Age At Onset, By Premorbid Social Adjustment

Premorbid social adjustment	Mean (SD) age at onset (yrs)		t-Value	df	P-Value
	Males	Females			
Good	35.2 (16.8)	42.5 (20.6)	−3.29	297	.001
Poor	26.8 (11.2)	36.6 (20.3)	−4.08	171	.000

95% CI=0.28–0.59), to have poor premorbid social (47% vs. 26%; RR=0.38; 95% CI=0.26–0.56) and work (47% vs. 33%; RR=0.55; 95% CI=0.38–0.81) adjustment; and to have had a diagnosable personality disorder prior to illness onset (24% vs. 11%; RR=0.39; 95% CI=0.24–0.66).

We proceeded to investigate gender differences in the early- and late-onset patients separately (see Tables 4.2a, b). It will be noted that significant differences between men and women remain for all the premorbid variables in the early-onset cases, but that later-onset men

TABLE 4.2a
Premorbid Social And Occupational Adjustment By Sex, For All Non-Affective Psychotics < 36 Years Age At Onset

Parameter	Male	Female	Risk ratio; 95% CI
Single*	139 (78%)	70 (59%)	0.40; 0.24–0.66
Poor work adjustment	105 (59%)	51 (43%)	0.53; 0.33–0.85
Poor social adjustment	100 (56%)	39 (33%)	0.38; 0.23–0.62
Personality disorder	52 (29%)	18 (15%)	0.44; 0.24–0.79

* Single=never married or cohabited.

Table 4.2b
Premorbid Social And Occupational Adjustment By Sex, For All Non-Affective
Psychotics › 35 Years Age At Onset Only

Parameter	Male	Female	Risk ratio; 95% CI
Single*	22 (36%)	39 (33%)	0.88; 0.46–1.70
Poor work adjustment	6 (10%)	27 (23%)	2.76; 1.07–7.12
Poor social adjustment	13 (21%)	21 (18%)	0.82; 0.38–1.79
Personality disorder	5 (3%)	8 (7%)	0.84; 0.26–2.68

* Single = never married or cohabited.

and women do not differ significantly in terms of these variables. In sum, it appears that it is early-onset males who are most impaired in their premorbid functioning, and that it is this group who contribute most to the variance between males and females overall.

To ascertain the most powerful independent associations with age at onset in males and females, we performed a logistic regression analysis. Using a step-up approach, we constructed logistic regression equations for males and females separately, and then combined. The "best fit" equations are shown in Tables 4.3a, b, and c. The influences of poor premorbid social adjustment and personality disorder disappeared once single marital status was controlled for, leaving single marital status and poor premorbid work adjustment as the main variables associated with early illness-onset. It will also be noted from Tables 4.3a and b that these factors operated in

TABLE 4.3a
Logistic Regression Parameters (Adjusted) With Age At Onset
As Dependent Variable, Males Only

Parameter	Exp B	Se B	P-Value
Single	0.21	0.35	.000
Poor work adjustment	0.09	0.47	.000

TABLE 4.3b
Logistic Regression Parameters (Adjusted) With Age At Onset
As Dependent Variable, Females Only

Parameter	Exp B	Se B	P-Value
Single	0.34	0.27	.000
Poor work adjustment	0.44	0.29	.006

TABLE 4.3c
Logistic Regression Parameters (Adjusted) With Age At Onset
As Dependent Variable, Both Sexes Combined

Parameter	Exp B	Se B	P-Value
Single	0.27	0.22	.000
Poor work adjustment	0.25	0.24	.000
Sex (female)	2.25	0.22	.002

the same manner for both men and women (i.e. there was no significant statistical interaction). In the combined male/female analysis (Table 4.3c), sex was found to be an independent predictor of early onset even after controlling for all other variables (although the strength of the association was marginally reduced).

Age-at-onset distribution curves

Figure 4.2 shows rates for DSM-III–R defined schizophrenia, by gender; DSM-III–R criteria were chosen as they are not restrictive in terms of age at onset. The curves for men and women are quite different from each

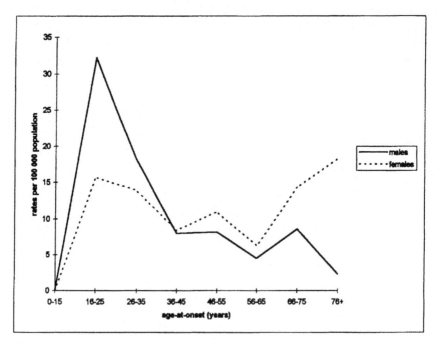

FIG. 4.2.   Rates for DSM-III–R schizophrenia, by gender.

other in shape. In those patients with an onset under 30 years, males predominated with an emphatic peak, whilst the distribution for females was flatter. In contrast, the patients with an onset after 60 years had a marked excess of females, with a late peak of incidence which was far less emphatic for males. In the mid-ages, females again predominated, with an incidence curve which was echoed by the males, although reaching a lower peak.

These data were subjected to an admixture analysis, using SKUMIX, to determine the best statistical fit for the distribution in men and women. Table 4.4 shows the results of these analyses. Males showed evidence of two age at onset distributions ($P = .004$), with modes at 21.4 years and 39.2 years. Females also showed evidence of two distributions ($P < .001$), with the suggestion of a third peak ($P = .06$). The modes of the three distributions in females were 22.4, 36.6, and 61.5 years.

DISCUSSION

The findings reported here, of a difference in the mean age at onset between men and women with non-affective functional psychotic disorders, recapitulates numerous prior reports of such differences. However, the sampling frame allows us to take prior reports a step further in that patients were selected independent of diagnosis or age at onset. The relatively large differential in onset in the current sample reflects our inclusion of patients with a very late onset of illness; such patients have been excluded from most previous studies.

We were able to confirm that the later onset of schizophrenia in women is not an artifact of diagnosis, in that the effect was robust to stringency of diagnosis. Of interest is the relatively high proportion of patients with a late onset of illness who fulfilled stringent diagnostic criteria for schizophrenia.

The effect of marital status on age at onset reported here point to married men and women having a later mean onset of illness. This is

TABLE 4.4
Admixture Analysis Of Age At Onset, Using SKUMIX

Sex	No. of groups	χ^2	Df	P-Value
Male	2 vs. 1	11.12	2	0.00
	3 vs. 2	1.52	2	0.47
Female	2 vs. 1	49.62	2	0.00
	3 vs. 2	5.44	2	0.06

hardly a surprising finding, and probably reflects a combination of better premorbid functioning in individuals with a later onset; a longer illness-free period in which to marry; and possibly some "protective" effect of marriage itself. When only single individuals were considered, the sex difference in onset disappeared. This is again in line with the notion that there is a severe early-onset form of illness associated with premorbid and psychosocial impairment. It is not as though women are free of risk for such an illness, merely that they are less likely to get it. In support of this conclusion, we found that, in terms of premorbid adjustment, it was males with an early onset of illness who fared worst, although early-onset females were also more impaired than their late-onset counterparts.

In defining the main contributions to age at onset, we found robust independent associations between early onset and single marital status, as well as poor premorbid work adjustment; these factors operated in much the same way for both men and women. Sex itself was found to be an independent predictor of early illness onset, even after controlling for other premorbid variables.

What is also clear from the current data is that the age at onset distribution curves for men and women with non-affective psychotic disorders are not isomorphic. Thus, it is not as though the curve for women is merely shifted to the right, as would be predicted by a simple explanation for the difference in onset in terms of some factor delaying onset in women. The different distributions demand a more sophisticated explanatory hypothesis. One possibility is that there are different forms of illness with different mean onset, to which males and females are differentially prone. This possibility is explored further in the following chapter.

CHAPTER FIVE

Subtypes of schizophrenia as expressions of wider dimensions of psychosis

This chapter describes a latent class classification of gender differences in schizophrenia and related disorders in the Camberwell Register sample of non-organic non-affective psychotic patients. Unlike previous attempts at similar factor analyses, the current study has the major methodological advantages of including all contacts of Camberwell residents with the psychiatric services, and not only those actually admitted to hospital. As described earlier, the study is catchment-area based, includes patients across all ages at onset, and the fact that it encompasses a very broad range of diagnostic groups, avoids conclusions being drawn about patients already preselected according to any specific set of diagnostic criteria. These methodological advantages are particularly pertinent to studies of gender differences in schizophrenia in that males, with a tendency to manifest a particularly severe form of schizophrenia, are overrepresented in hospitalised samples and in groups fulfilling stringent criteria for the illness.

As outlined in Chapter 4, and already confirmed in this epidemiologically based sample, males with schizophrenia have a mean onset at an earlier age than do females. Furthermore, the age-at-onset distribution differs markedly for men and women. This has profound implications for any theory aimed at explaining gender differences in schizophrenia (see Castle & Murray, 1993). One possibility is that some factor associated with being female serves to delay the onset of the illness. The factor to attract most attention has been oestrogen; thus, the oestrogen hypothesis proposes that during the reproductive years, women are somehow "protected" by the antidopaminergic action of oestrogens, and that the slight peak in the incidence of female schizophrenia in the 46–55 year age range is the result of removal of such protection at the menopause (see Hafner et al., 1991; Riecher-Rossler & Hafner, 1993).

Whilst clinical, epidemiological, and animal studies confirm an effect of oestrogens on dopamine pathways, and hence by inference psychopathology, the oestrogen hypothesis in its simplest form cannot account for the extent of gender differences seen in the functional psychoses. The limitations of the oestrogen hypothesis in this regard have been detailed elsewhere (Castle, Abel, Takei, & Murray, 1995). In particular, a theory which emphasises the role of pubertal and post-pubertal oestrogen production cannot account for the following: (1) males predominate in those few patients whose onset of schizophrenia antedates puberty; (2) premorbid social and occupational dysfunction are more commonly features of male than female schizophrenia; (3) premorbid IQ is lower in males, but not females, who later develop schizophrenia; (4) males overall manifest more "negative" schizophrenic symptoms than their female counterparts; and (5) females far exceed males among cases with a very late onset of illness (i.e. long past the menopause).

An alternative explanation is that the gender differences in age at onset are a clue to subtypes of schizophrenia to which men and women are differentially prone (see Castle & Murray, 1991; Goldstein, Santangelo, Simpson, & Tsuang, 1990; Murray, O'Callaghan, Castle, & Lewis, 1992). Specifically, we have suggested that males are particularly likely to manifest a severe, early-onset form of illness akin to Kraepelin's "dementia praecox"; some females with schizophrenia do have this form of illness, but they are relatively few in number. A milder form of illness with generally later onset and with links to affective disorder, is female predominated. Finally, there may be a very late-onset (generally >60 years) form of schizophrenia-like psychosis in which there is a marked excess of females.

To investigate whether a typology of schizophrenia based on gender could be derived from this catchment-area sample, we used a latent class analytic approach. These data are presented in more detail in Castle et al. (1994) and Sham, Castle, Wessely, Farmer, and Murray (1996).

Latent class analysis, a form of factor analysis, involves the construction of latent variables to explain the associations between observed or manifest variables, dealing with categorical manifest variables and assuming a categorical latent variable (Green, 1951; Lazarsfeld & Henry, 1968). In the latent class analysis described here, the example of Goldstein et al. (1990) was followed, in using simultaneous latent class models (Clogg & Goodman, 1985), with gender-specific latent classes. These models are specified by restricting the conditional probability of being male at unity in some latent classes, and at zero in others. Interest is focused on the number of latent classes in each gender, and the extent to which the latent classes of the two genders correspond to each other. A sequence of latent class models were fitted, ranging from one to three latent classes per gender, with and without the restrictions of total homogeneity on the within-class conditional probabilities. The program MLLSA (Maximum Likelihood Latent Structure Analysis) developed by Clogg (1977) was used throughout.

VARIABLES CONSIDERED: LATENT CLASS ANALYSIS

The variables for the analysis were chosen to provide a coverage of aetiological (putatively genetic or environmental), premorbid, and phenomenological parameters, as well as gender and age at onset. The variables were: (1) family history of schizophrenia in first- or second-degree relatives (FH); (2) winter birth, i.e. December to April (WB); (3) poor premorbid social adjustment (SA); (4) restricted affect (RA); (5) persecutory delusions (PD); (6) dysphoria (DS); (7) early onset, i.e. 25 years or younger (EO); and (8) male sex (MS). The variables are defined in OCCPI 2.5. As such, the variables approximate those used by Goldstein et al. (1990).

There were 447 patients with non-affective functional psychosis, for whom all the manifest variables for use in stage 1 of the latent class analysis had been recorded. The distributions of the eight chosen manifest variables are given in Table 5.1. Summary statistics for pairwise relationships are given in Table 5.2, with the size of association being measured by product moment (Pearson's) correlation coefficients, and the statistical significance assessed by chi-squared tests for 2×2 tables. The most significant positive associations were between male sex and poor premorbid social adjustment, early onset and poor premorbid social adjustment, and the most significant negative association was between early onset and paranoid delusions. To these data, the following six latent class models were fitted:

M1. One latent class per gender, with total homogeneity.
M2. One latent class per gender, totally unconstrained.
M3. Two latent classes per gender, with total homogeneity.
M4. Two latent classes per gender, totally unconstrained.
M5. Three latent classes per gender, with total homogeneity.
M6. Three latent classes per gender, totally unconstrained.

Table 5.1
The Distributions Of The Manifest Variables

	Present (1)	Absent (0)
Family history (FH)	35	412
Restricted affect (RA)	48	399
Persecutory delusion (PD)	346	101
Poor social adjustment (SA)	165	282
Dysphoria (DS)	213	234
Early onset (EO)	166	281
Winter birth (WB)	196	251
Male sex (MS)	227	220

(From Castle et al., 1994. Reprinted with the permission of Cambridge University Press.)

TABLE 5.2
Pairwise Product Moment Correlations Of The Manifest Variables

FH	1							
RA	.060	1						
PD	.038	−.020	1					
SA	.053	.169***	−.086*	1				
DS	−.095*	.045	.044	.069	1			
EO	.086	.197***	−.282****	.237****	.027	1		
WB	.078	−.030	−.008	−.069	.015	−.017	1	
MS	−.046	.183***	−.050	.215****	−.145**	.164***	.022	1
	FH	RA	PD	SA	DS	EO	WB	MS

* $P<.1$; ** $P<.01$; *** $P<.001$; **** $P<.0001$ (chi-squared test of independence with Yate's correction).
(From Castle et al., 1994. Reprinted with the permission of Cambridge University Press.)

Two global measures of goodness-of-fit, the Pearson (χ^2) and likelihood ratio (L^2) chi-squared statistics, and their associated degrees of freedom (df), were obtained for each model using MLLSA (Table 5.3). Both χ^2 and L^2 were very large for M1, which was therefore excluded from further consideration. In any event, the clinical interpretation of M1, that there is one disorder identical in the two genders, is contrary to the literature on gender difference in schizophrenia reviewed above.

The interpretation of M2 is that there are two subtypes, one of which occurs solely in men, and the other in women. In contrast, M3 suggests the existence of two subtypes which occur in men and women in different proportions. These two models differ only slightly in df, but enormously in both χ^2 and L^2, with M3 providing a much better fit to the data. M2 was therefore excluded from further consideration.

TABLE 5.3
Global Goodness Of Fit Test Statistics For
Models 1–6

Model	χ^2	L^2	df
M1	465.18	325.85	247
M2	419.39	265.42	240
M3	264.18	222.99	238
M4	250.41	176.96	225
M5	245.34	204.51	230
M6	260.68	157.67	214

(From Castle et al., 1994. Reprinted with the permission of Cambridge University Press.)

The next comparison is between M3 and M4. The interpretation of M4, like that of M2, suggests that there is no relationship between the subtypes in men and women. Here the evidence from χ^2 and L^2 as to whether M3 or M4 is the best statistical fit is not consistent; the difference in L^2 (46.03) is significant, suggesting M4 to be a better fit.

M5 postulates the existence of three subtypes which occur in both genders in different proportions. The parameter restrictions in M5 make it more parsimonious than M4 (by 5 *df*), so that a slightly worse goodness-of-fit is acceptable for M5. However, the evidence from χ^2 and L^2 point to opposite directions; χ^2 favours M5 while L^2 favours M4.

Finally, M6 is a model with three subtypes in men and three unrelated subtypes in women. Comparing M5 and M6, which differ by 16 *df*, the difference in χ^2 is 15.34 in favour of M5, but the difference in L^2 is 46.84 in favour of M6. Hence, the global goodness-of-fit statistics are not consistent with each other, a reflection of the large number of cells in the contingency table, many of which would be expected to be empty. Thus, instead of relying solely on global test statistics the expected cell counts and residuals were examined, revealing that the fit of M3 was poorer that of the other three models. However, the degrees of freedom for M4, M5, and M6, which fit the data almost equally well, are 225, 230, and 214 respectively, showing that M6 is far less parsimonious than the other two models. M4 and M5 are statistically very similar.

Table 5.4 shows that M4 is characterised by the existence of a subtype (classes 1 and 3) with a high frequency of positive family history, early onset, restricted affect, and poor premorbid adjustment, and a male to female ratio of 2:1. Interestingly, within this type, more males (class 1) than females (class 3) have restricted affect and poor premorbid adjustment, but more females than males have a positive family history of schizophrenia. The second possible subtype (classes 2 and 4) has a

TABLE 5.4
Parameter Estimates For M4

Model 4	Males		Females	
	X = 1	X = 2	X = 3	X = 4
P(X)	.22	.29	.11	.38
P(FH = 1|X)	.11	.03	.14	.08
P(RA = 1|X)	.30	.06	.13	.03
P(PD = 1|X)	.65	.83	.43	.90
P(SA = 1|X)	.72	.29	.44	.21
P(DS = 1|X)	.50	.34	.56	.55
P(EO = 1|X)	.78	.20	1.0	.08
P(WB = 1|X)	.36	.51	.53	.40
P(MS = 1|X)	(1)	(1)	(0)	(0)

The latent categorical variable, X, takes values 1, 2, 3, 4, each representing a latent class. The parameters P(X) are the probabilities of the different values of X, i.e. the probabilities of the latent classes. The parameters P(FH = 1|X), P(RA = 1|X), etc., are the conditional probabilities of the manifest variable taking a value of 1, given the value of the latent categorical variable, i.e. the within-class conditional probabilities of the manifest variables. The parameters in brackets, i.e. the conditional probabilities of being male within the latent classes, are fixed constants.

(From Castle et al., 1994. Reprinted with the permission of Cambridge University Press.)

higher frequency of persecutory delusions, and a female excess. The two subtypes do not differ much with regard to dysphoria. Confusingly, winter birth appears to be more frequent in classes 2 and 3 than in classes 1 and 4, i.e. it appears to be more frequent in the males of the second subtype and the females of the first subtype.

M5 is easier to interpret (Table 5.5). First, there is a subtype (classes 1 and 4; henceforth type A) with a high frequency of positive family history, early onset, restricted affect, and poor premorbid adjustment, and a male to female ratio of just over 2:1. This subtype is very similar to the first subtype in M4. The second subtype (classes 2 and 5; type B) has a high frequency of persecutory delusions and winter birth, a low frequency of early onset, and a male to female ratio of about unity. This subtype is similar to the second subtype in M4. The third subtype (classes 3 and 6; type C) has a very high frequency of dysphoria and persecutory delusions, a very low frequency of family history of schizophrenia and restricted affect, and very few men.

Thus, M5 can be considered a special case of M4. Because of the advantages outlined above, this is the model which was taken forward to stage 2 of the latent class analysis.

TABLE 5.5
Parameter Estimates For M5

	Males			Females		
Model 5	X = 1	X = 2	X = 3	X = 4	X = 5	X = 6
P(X)	.29	.22	.00	.13	.23	.13
P(FH = 1|X)	.10	.07	.01	.10	.07	.01
P(RA = 1|X)	.22	.03	.00	.22	.03	.00
P(PD = 1|X)	.61	.88	.93	.61	.88	.93
P(SA = 1|X)	.60	.20	.23	.60	.20	.23
P(DS = 1|X)	.50	.31	.98	.50	.31	.98
P(EO = 1|X)	.74	.09	.16	.74	.09	.16
P(WB = 1|X)	.41	.51	.28	.41	.51	.28
P(MS = 1|X)	(1)	(1)	(1)	(0)	(0)	(0)

The latent categorical variable, X, takes values 1, 2, 3, 4, 5, 6 each representing a latent class. The parameters P(X) are the probabilities of the different values of X, i.e. the probabilities of the latent classes. The parameters P(FH = 1|X), P(RA = 1|X), etc., are the conditional probabilities of the manifest variable taking a value of 1, given the value of the latent categorical variable, i.e. the within-class conditional probabilities of the manifest variables. The parameters in brackets, i.e. the conditional probabilities of being male within the latent classes, are fixed constants.

(From Castle et al., 1994. Reprinted with the permission of Cambridge University Press.)

STAGE 2 OF THE LATENT CLASS ANALYSIS

Each of the 447 subjects was assigned to one of the classes in M5, and correlations explored between the type of illness and a range of family history, premorbid, phenomenological, and treatment response character- istics (variables as defined in OCCPI). All variables were dichotomous, being scored 1 if the characteristic was present and 0 if absent.

The correlations are shown in Tables 5.6a–c. Among "premorbid" variables, type A is characterised by a relatively high frequency of obstetric complications, developmental problems, premorbid personality disorder, single marital status, poor premorbid work adjustment, positive offending history, and long prodromal phase. Indeed, all positive "premorbid" features were commoner in type A than in types B or C, with the exception of family history of psychiatric disorder other than schizo- phrenia (mostly affective disorder), which was commonest in type C.

In terms of the "phenomenological" variables, the subtypes did not differ significantly in first rank symptoms, auditory hallucinations, or bizarre delusions. This is to be expected since these are the symptoms typical of schizophrenia. Type A had the highest frequencies of thought disorder, negative symptoms, "manic" symptomatology, inappropriate

TABLE 5.6a
Comparing The Subtypes In Terms Of "Premorbid" Variables

Characteristic	Percentage present			P-value
	Type A (N = 168)	Type B (N = 175)	Type C (N = 83)	
Family history of other psychiatric disorders	32.0	20.9	36.8	.0100
Alcoholism in parents	11.8	9.3	3.4	.0863
Obstetric complications	14.9	3.4	2.4	.0042
Developmental problems	11.0	5.9	2.1	.1007
Premorbid personality disorder	31.5	8.8	9.2	<.0001
Single marital status	86.5	39.6	33.3	<.0001
Poor premorbid work adjustment	61.2	25.4	29.9	<.0001
Unemployed	66.3	59.1	51.7	.0656
Forensic history	42.6	22.6	12.9	<.0001
Prodromal phase	62.4	50.8	44.8	.0130

TABLE 5.6b
Comparing The Subtypes In Terms Of "Phenomenological" Variables

Characteristic	Percentage present			P-value
	Type A (N = 168)	Type B (N = 175)	Type C (N = 83)	
Depressive symptomatology	64.0	40.7	86.2	<.0001
Manic symptomatology	39.3	25.3	31.0	.0165
Unspecified affective symptoms	34.3	17.6	54.0	<.0001
First-rank symptoms	57.3	53.8	52.9	.7268
Thought disorder	37.6	25.3	12.6	.0001
Negative symptoms	51.1	29.1	21.8	<.0001
Paranoid delusions	73.6	89.6	85.1	.0003
Auditory hallucinations	62.9	69.8	75.9	.0883
Inappropriate affect	21.3	8.8	13.8	.0034
Bizarre delusions	25.3	21.4	17.2	.3194
Bizarre behaviour	53.4	36.8	51.7	.0037
Catatonia	10.7	3.8	1.1	.0025

TABLE 5.6c
Comparing The Subtypes In Terms Of "Treatment Response" Variables

Characteristic	Percentage present			P-value
	Type A (N = 168)	Type B (N = 175)	Type C (N = 83)	
Response to neuroleptic	71.3	77.5	85.1	0435

Note: Tables 5.6a,b, & c reprinted, with permission, from Sham et al., 1996.

affect, bizarre behaviour, and catatonia. The high rate of "manic" symptoms probably reflects the broad definition of "mania" that was employed; for example, "distractibility", one of its constituent symptoms, could also be a sign of acute schizophrenic psychosis. Type B had the highest frequency of paranoid delusions. Type C had the highest frequencies of depressive symptomatology and unspecified affective symptoms. Differences in response to neuroleptic treatment were only marginally significant, with type A being the least and type C the most frequently responsive.

THE SUBTYPES

Thus, our results suggest three types of illness, viz.:

(1) The first subtype, which we term *neurodevelopmental*, is represented by classes 1 and 4 of M5, and characterised by early onset, poor premorbid adjustment, restricted affect, and male preponderance. This form is associated with premorbid social maladjustment, personality disorder, and positive offending history, and has a high frequency of restricted and inappropriate affect, negative features, thought disorder, and catatonia. It also showed the highest rates of a family history of schizophrenia and of a history of obstetric complications, aetiological factors which have been implicated in the neurodevelopmental abnormality in schizophrenia (see Murray et al., 1992). Winter birth, on the other hand, does not appear to be excessively common. Thus, the neurodevelopmental form of illness with its male predominance, early onset of illness, and poor outcome has all the hallmarks of what Kraepelin termed "dementia praecox". Furthermore, a separate longitudinal study of this "Kraepelinian" type of schizophrenia has shown a more severe course for such patients than for their non-Kraepelinian counterparts (Keefe et al., 1996).

We (Castle & Murray, 1991) have suggested that the male propensity to such an illness should be considered in the context of the broader literature on sex differences in the brain, expressly the vulnerability of males to all neurodevelopmental illnesses (e.g. autism). This debate will increasingly be informed by the burgeoning literature on differences in the development, structure, and function of male and female brains (e.g. Ames, 1991; Kimura, 1992; Murphy et al., 1996; Seeman, 1989; Taylor, 1969).

It should be emphasised that none of the variables included in this set of analyses are direct measures of structural brain abnormalities, and thus the proposed "neurodevelopmental" aetiology is presumptive. However, some support for this assumption comes from studies showing an association between poor premorbid functioning (and negative symptomatology) and structural brain abnormalities in schizophrenia (see Orel et al., 1991; Pearlson et al., 1985, 1989; Weinberger, Cannon-Spoor, Potkin, & Wyatt, 1980), as well as the fact that schizophrenic males (and expressly young males) appear most likely to show such abnormalities on neuroimaging investigations. Thus, Cowell et al. (1996) who carried a recent MRI study designed to investigate sex differences in the relationships between brain and behaviour did indeed conclude their findings "suggest that aspects of the neuropathological basis for some symptoms in schizophrenia may be sexually dimorphic."

Similarly, although we did not have systematic neuropsychological measures, a number of studies have shown that preschizophrenics, especially males, have lower childhood intelligence than their siblings and peers (Aylward, Walker, & Betts, 1984). Furthermore, lower childhood IQ predicts poor outcome as was shown by Russell, Munro, Jones, Hemsley, and Murray (1997), who examined WAIS scores for children seen at the Maudsley Child Psychiatry services who later went on to develop adult schizophrenia; not only did these children show lower than expected IQ, but low IQ predicted chronic illness and negative symptoms in adult life.

This is one example of a more general finding: childhood developmental deficit is not only a risk factor for the *emergence* of schizophrenia especially in males, but is also an important risk factor for illness *persistence* (Stoffelmayr, Dillavou, & Hunter, 1983). Thus, two prospective four–six year studies (Breier, Schreiber, & Dyer, 1992; Verdoux et al., 1996) which examined childhood function using the scale of Philips (1953) found a similar association between poor premorbid adjustment and bad outcome of illness, especially in terms of negative symptoms and unemployment.

(2) Classes 2 and 5 of M5 ("*paranoid*" subtype) are characterised by later onset, paranoid delusions, and an almost equal sex ratio. It is generally a milder illness with much less restricted affect, negative features and thought disorder. It is proposed that these classes represent a "paranoid" subtype, similar to the paranoid subtype of Tsuang and Winokur (1974), and to the *P* cluster of Farmer, McGuffin, and Spitznagel (1983). In line with these previous studies, the "paranoid group" showed a lower familial risk for schizophrenia. The season of birth effect in this group, with 52% of patients having a date of birth between December and April, is intriguing. In an extensive review of the literature, Bradbury and Miller (1985) found no consistent schizophrenic subtype to be more prone to the seasonality effect. However, Opler, Kay, Rosado, and Lindenmayer (1984) and Takei et al. (1992) reported more winter birth effect in patients with later onset of illness.

(3) Classes 3 and 6 of M5 ("*schizoaffective*" subtype) are characterised by dysphoria, paranoid delusions, a negligible familial risk of schizophrenia, and an absence of men. We concluded that these classes represent

a "schizoaffective" subtype. Previous attempts at subtyping schizophrenia have not identified such a group of patients. This may be due to patient selection: while the current analyses involved the broad ICD-9 conception of schizophrenia and related disorders, others (e.g. Tsuang & Winokur, 1974) have used restrictive criteria (e.g. those of Feighner et al., 1972) which could have excluded such patients.

On the other hand, studies which examine psychosis as a whole report that the strongest argument against qualitative differences between schizophrenia and affective disorder is the existence of intermediate forms, the so-called schizoaffective disorders (Kasanin, 1933). Not only is their phenomenology intermediate but the course of these disorders is also intermediate: more benign than in schizophrenia, but worse than in affective psychosis. For example, Tsuang and Dempsey (1979), in a 30–40-year longitudinal study, showed that outcome for a group of 85 patients exhibiting both affective and schizophrenic features was significantly poorer than for a group of 325 patients with affective disorders, and significantly better than for a group of 200 schizophrenia patients. Similar findings were reported by Brockington and colleagues (1980a,b), Marneros and collaborators (1989, 1990), Coryell and colleagues (1990a,b), and Maj and Perris (1990).

Our delineation of a schizoaffective subtype is in line with the findings of gender differences outlined in Chapter 4, and are compatible with the suggestion that some females, who are diagnosed as having schizophrenia, have a form of illness related to affective disorder in aetiology. In support of this notion is the fact that the patients in this group often had a family history of psychiatric disorders other than schizophrenia (most of which would have been affective disorders). In one of the few published studies to compare schizophrenic patients with and without a family history of affective disorder, Kendler and Hays (1983) found that those patients with a family history of depression were more likely than those without such a history to develop a depressive syndrome during follow-up. Also, Owen, Lewis, and Murray (1989) found that schizophrenic patients with a family history of affective disorder were less likely to have structural brain abnormalities than other schizophrenic patients.

THE RELATIONSHIP OF SUBTYPES TO DIMENSIONS OF PSYCHOSIS

How do the above findings concerning typology within schizophrenia fit in with the dimensional concept of psychosis outlined in the introduction? How can there be both heterogeneity within schizophrenia and continuity without schizophrenia? The most parsimonious explanation of the subtypes that we elicited is that they represent the expression within the artificially defined category of schizophrenia of dimensional factors which operate across psychosis.

The neurodevelopmental dimension

Our neurodevelopmental subtype of schizophrenia can be seen as one end of a continuum of impairment which stretches across psychosis. For example, Jones et al. (1994a) showed that delayed milestones, speech difficulties, and lower IQ in childhood are risk factors for later schizophrenia in a birth cohort of nearly 5000 children born in the UK one week in 1946; two-thirds of those who developed schizophrenia were male. In the same cohort, we (Van Os, Jones, Lewis, Wadsworth, & Murray, 1997a) later found an excess of similar premorbid handicaps in subjects who went on to develop chronic depression. The development deviance was similar to, but generally less severe than, that found in preschizophrenics, but most interestingly it predicted later depression only in females. These findings raise the possibility that neurodevelopmental impairment in childhood is modulated by gender to increase the later risk of schizophrenia in males and chronic depression in females.

Furthermore, the association noted earlier between premorbid function and outcome of adult disorder is not specific to schizophrenia. A large number of studies have shown a similar relationship in unipolar, bipolar, and schizoaffective disorders (Brodaty et al., 1993; Coryell et al., 1990c; Deister & Marneros, 1993; Duggan, Lee, & Murray, 1990; Harder et al., 1990). The study of Werry, McClelland, and Chard (1991) illustrates this particularly well, being based on incident and representative cases of adolescent-onset psychosis (DSM-III schizophrenia ($n = 30$) and bipolar disorder ($n = 23$)) collected in a defined catchment area. Abnormal premorbid adjustment, using DSM-III–R major divisions of personality disorder on a four-point severity scale, emerged as the best predictor for poor five-year outcome in both schizophrenic and bipolar cases, but more so in schizophrenia. Overall, premorbid adaptational functioning explained 7% of occupational functioning, 10% of peer relationships, and 4% of adaptational functioning.

One could speculate that prenatal exposure to some winter-born virus such as influenza could cause some subtle brain abnormality which only becomes functionally manifest in association with the effects of advancing age. In this context it is of interest that prenatal exposure to influenza has been associated not only with later schizophrenia but also in one study with Parkinson's disease. It is clear, however, that our typology does not adequately account for patients with a very late-onset form of illness (> 60 years). This group of patients is discussed in Chapter 6, and are contrasted with their very early-onset "dementia praecox" counterparts.

The affective dimension

It is not difficult to see that our schizoaffective type is merely an extension into "schizophrenic territory" of a factor which operates very obviously within affective disorder. The literature offers little support for the view that there are qualitative differences in outcome between schizophrenia and manic-depressive psychosis. Although the outcome of schizophrenia is, on average, worse than of affective disorder, considerable overlap exists, with many schizophrenic patients, particularly females and those with acute onset, showing good outcome and many affective disorder patients having poor outcome (Lee & Murray, 1988; McGlashan, 1984; Murray et al., 1992).

A paranoid dimension?

It is also easy to see the paranoid subtype as an expression within schizophrenia of a dimension which also operates outside it; perhaps in this case the archetype condition is paranoid psychosis. The excess winter births of members of this subtype is of interest in view of the fact that a similar winter birth excess has been reported by a number of investigators in atypical and affective as well as schizophrenic psychosis.

CONCLUSION

The analyses presented here are based on a large representative catchment-area sample of patients not preselected according to age at onset or any specific set of diagnostic criteria. Different analytical approaches suggested that gender differences in the sample can be interpreted in terms of a differential susceptibility of men and women to three subtypes of schizophrenia.

We do not consider that the demonstration of these three subtypes is in any way contradictory to the view outlined in the introduction to this book that psychosis should be seen as a continuum. On the contrary, we regard these idealised subtypes as the expressions within the artificial category of schizophrenia of dimensions which operate to a greater or lesser extent across psychosis.

CHAPTER SIX

Late-onset schizophrenia

We turn now to a consideration of those patients with a first manifestation of a schizophrenia-like illness in late life. Some of the data presented here have been published elsewhere (Castle & Murray, 1993; Castle, Wessely, Howard, & Murray, 1997; Howard, Castle, Wessely, & Murray, 1993): this chapter serves to integrate and expand those publications in the broader context of this book. First, a brief overview of the relevant literature is provided (based on Castle et al., 1997).

It was Kraepelin (1896) who used the term "paraphrenia" to describe those non-affective non-organic psychoses not subsumed under his label of "dementia praecox". As outlined in Chapters 4 and 5, dementia praecox defines a group of patients with an early onset of illness, premorbid dysfunction, and severe course; most of the individuals to fulfil such criteria are male. We have detailed in Chapter 5 our view that such individuals have a neurodevelopmental disorder.

In contrast, Kraepelin's paraphrenia cases (systematica, expansiva, confabulans, and phantastica) generally had a later-onset (around 40 years) more benign form of illness with better preservation of personality and less disturbance of volition; delusional content was generally more believable, and reasoning intact apart from those areas impinged upon by the delusional beliefs (see Addonizio, 1995). Mayer (1921) followed up 78 cases assigned to the paraphrenia category by Kraepelin, and found the majority did show some decline in general social functioning and increase in paranoia over the years. Mayer concluded that the paraphrenia cases merely reflected a later onset form of dementia praecox (by now the Bleulerian term "schizophrenia" had been adopted). This view became widely held in Europe and, despite Bleuler's continued reference to "the group of schizophrenias", European psychiatry tended to treat all schizophrenia-like psychoses as one disease category, irrespective of age at onset.

Roth (1955) resurrected the term paraphrenia (actually "late para-phrenia"), but somewhat confusingly used it to describe a very late-onset (>60 years) group with florid paranoid delusions, often with a well-organised theme, with or without auditory hallucinations, and with generally good preservation of personality. Roth showed that patients with this disorder had a very much better outcome than dementia patients. Kay and Roth (1961) subsequently performed a follow-up of 99 such cases, and their delineation of a late-onset group with female preponderance, low marital rates, low fertility, social isolation, and paranoid personality attributes, cemented the late paraphrenia concept in European psychiatry. Thus, ICD-9 (WHO, 1978) had a category of "paraphrenia", akin to Roth's original description of late paraphrenia. This has been dropped from ICD-10 (WHO, 1993), despite spirited protests from some workers (e.g. Almeida, Howard, Forstl, & Levy, 1992; Munro, 1991), who argue that the dissimilarities of such cases from those with an early onset make such a separate category useful.

The North American tradition has been very different, with major fluctuations in the conception of what constitutes "schizophrenia". The overinclusiveness of the American use of the term was delineated clearly in the US/UK diagnostic project (Cooper et al., 1972), and the subsequent definition of schizophrenia in the third revision of the *Diagnostic and Statistical Manual* (APA, 1980) was very narrow, including a preclusion of the diagnosis being made if onset of illness was after the age of 44 years. This stipulation has been removed in subsequent editions of the *Manual* (DSM-III–R, DSM-IV).

The term "paranoia" was also used by Kraepelin, to define a chronic psychotic condition with an encapsulated delusional system in the setting of well preserved personality (see Munro, 1991). This term also fell into disuse after Kolle (1931) found that a proportion of such cases showed a schizophrenia-like deterioration with time. However, a small group of patients with longstanding delusions do not show such deterioration, and such patients are defined in DSM-IV as "delusional (paranoid) disorder".

Given all this confusion, and the paucity of systematic population-based studies of non-affective psychoses in later life, we used the Camberwell Register sample to investigate these patients directly. We define the epidemiology (incidence, age-at-onset distribution, gender distribution) of such cases in a sample neither biased by hospital admission, nor preselected according to any particular set of diagnostic criteria for schizophrenia; also, we did not use any arbitrary age-at-onset cut-off. We also compared the phenomenology, premorbid functioning, and aetiological parameters (family history, obstetric complications, etc.) in those patients with a very early (< 25 years) and those with a very late (> 60 years) onset disorder.

THE CURRENT STUDY

Incidence rates

Figure 6.1 shows annual incidence rates for broadly defined schizophrenia and related disorders, as well as for those individuals fulfilling DSM-III–R criteria for schizophrenia. The DSM-III–R rates were adjusted for missing case records using the appropriate proportion of patients in the total sample fulfilling DSM-III–R criteria in each 10-year age at onset band. The distribution by age at onset was much the same irrespective of stringency of diagnosis. The highest rates were in the 16–25 year age group, with a slight second peak in the 46–55 year group, and a third (more emphatic) peak in the over-60s. The wide confidence limits for the later-onset patients is a reflection of the relatively small number of patients in this group.

Very early vs. very late-onset cases

Of the total 477 cases included in this set of analyses, 192 (40%) had an illness onset before they reached 25 years ("very early onset": 97 (20%) before 21 years, and 95 (20%) between 21 and 25 years). At the other end of the age spectrum, 72 cases (16%) had their first manifestation of illness after 60 years ("very late onset": 16 (3.5%) 60–65 years; 18 (3.5%) 66–70 years; 15 (3%) 71–75 years; 13 (2.5%) 76–80 years; and 10 (2%) over 80 years). Of the very early-onset group, 61% were male, compared to 24% of those with a very late onset (RR = 5.04; 95% CI = 2.73–9.35). The very early-onset patients were also more likely to be of African-Caribbean ethnicity (40% vs. 4%), a reflection of the changing sociodemographic patterns of Camberwell over the years, as detailed in Chapter 2.

A comparison of the very early- and very late-onset patients in terms of DSM-III–R criteria is shown in Table 6.1. The results reinforce the conclusions made above regarding very late-onset patients having a severe and florid disorder which fulfil stringent DSM-III–R criteria for schizophrenia (around one-third of the very early-onset cases vs. over half of those with onset after 60 years). As anticipated, very late-onset patients were more likely than their early-onset counterparts to meet criteria for delusional disorder (11.1% vs. 6.3%).

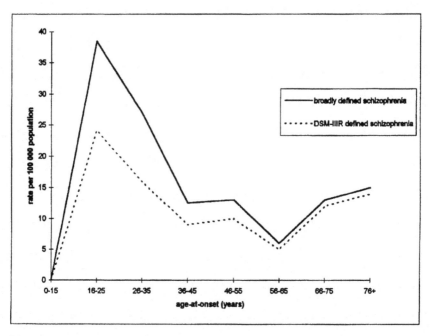

FIG. 6.1. First-contact rates for broadly defined and DSM-III-R defined schizophrenia.

Phenomenological parameters

The data on diagnostic criteria are somewhat misleading, in that a closer analysis of phenomenological variables revealed distinct differences between patients with an onset before 25 years, and those with first manifestation after 60 years of age. The differences are detailed in Table 6.2 (all ratings as in OCCPI 2.5). Specifically, formal thought disorder, passivity phenomena, thought interference, and negative symptoms (paucity of thought/speech, restricted affect) were more common in patients with an onset of illness under 25 years of age, while persecutory delusions, expressly in an elaborately organised form, and any form of auditory hallucination were more common in the very late-onset group. Indeed, the only symptoms not significantly differently distributed between these two groups of patients were delusional perception, bizarre delusions, and delusions of reference.

Although 98% of our very late-onset cases had delusions of a persecutory nature, in 22% these involved machines, x-rays, or other special means by which the persecutors tormented their victims. Nearly half of the cases reported so-called "partition" delusions (see Howard et al., 1992), where patients believed that people, objects, gases, or radiation

TABLE 6.1
Early- And Late-Onset Patients: Diagnosis According To DSM-III–R Criteria

	Atypical psychosis	Schizo-phreniform disorder	Schizo-phrenia	Delusional disorder
Early-onset patients (<25 yr)	44 (23%)	19 (10%)	71 (37%)	12 (6.3%)
Late-onset patients (>60 yr)	11 (15%)	11 (15%)	40 (56%)	8 (11%)

(Reprinted, with permission, from Castle et al., 1997.)

could enter their abode through objectively impermeable barriers. The majority of patients with a very late-onset disorder manifested one or more form of hallucination: 85% auditory, 22% visual, 10% olfactory, and 17% somatic.

Premorbid and aetiological comparisons

In terms of premorbid parameters, patients with an onset of illness after 60 years of age fared better than their very early-onset counterparts. The very early- and very late-onset groups differed markedly with respect to premorbid functioning, with 57% of the former but only 9% of the latter

TABLE 6.2a
Prevalence Of Symptoms More Common In Early-Onset Patients (< 25 yr)

	% in early-onset patients (<25 yr) (n=192)	% in late-onset patients (>60 yr) (n=72)	Risk ratio; 95% CI
Positive formal thought disorder	28.4	1.4	0.04; 0.00–0.30
Negative formal thought disorder	14.2	0.0	0.85; 0.81–0.91
Inappropriate affect	21.6	4.3	0.16; 0.05–0.54
Restricted affect	17.9	0.0	0.82; 0.79–0.88
Passivity delusions	29.3	9.8	0.26; 0.11–0.60
Catatonia	12.1	0.0	0.87; 0.83–0.92
Primary delusions other than delusional perception	16.8	2.8	0.14; 0.03–0.61
Thought insertion	16.8	1.4	0.07; 0.01–0.52
Thought withdrawal	10.0	1.4	0.13; 0.02–0.97
Grandiose delusions	22.1	8.5	0.32; 0.13–0.81

(Reprinted, with permission, from Castle et al., 1997.)

TABLE 6.2b
Prevalence Of Symptoms More Common In Late-Onset Patients (> 60 yr)

	% in early-onset patients (< 25 yr) (n = 192)	% in late-onset patients (> 60 yr) (n = 72)	Risk ratio; 95% CI
Persecutory delusions	61.6	93.1	8.25; 3.17–21.43
Organised delusions	12.6	55.7	8.65; 4.57–16.35
Widespread delusions	42.9	70.4	3.17; 1.77–4.67
Third-person auditory hallucinations	28.9	41.7	1.74; 1.01–13.06
Accusatory or abusive voices	43.7	67.6	2.63; 1.48–4.67
Persecutory delusions with hallucinations	48.9	76.1	2.54; 1.37–4.70

(Reprinted, with permission, from Castle et al., 1997.)

judged to have had poor premorbid work adjustment (RR = 0.07; 95% CI = 0.03–0.17). Similarly, 21% of very late- vs. 50% of very early-onset patients were rated (OCCPI criteria) as having shown poor premorbid social adjustment (RR = 0.27; 95% CI = 0.14–0.51). Consonant with this finding, 67% of the very late-onset group were currently or had been married, the proportion in the very early-onset group being only 15% (RR = 0.08; 95% CI = 0.04–0.17).

In exploring those aetiological parameters implicated in the aetiology of schizophrenia, as detailed in Chapter 5, the patients with an onset of illness below 25 had, in comparison with their late-onset counterparts, a higher rate of obstetric complications (14.1% vs. 4.5%; RR = 0.29; 95% CI = 0.03–2.29), and developmental difficulty (11.9% vs. 0%; RR = 0.88; 95% CI = 0.83–0.94). In terms of familial loading, early-onset cases were more likely to have a positive family history of schizophrenia (10.2% vs. 2.9%; RR = 0.26; 95% CI = 0.06–1.16), but not of other serious psychiatric disorder (30.6% vs. 23.5%; RR = 0.69; 95% CI = 0.37–1.32).

Further characteristics of the late-onset cases

A number of other parameters are reportedly associated with late-onset psychosis, including premorbid paranoid personality traits, social isolation, and sensory impairment (reviewed by Castle & Howard, 1992). However, almost all previous studies have been based on samples biased in terms of severity (usually hospitalised patients only). Our sampling frame enabled us to assess such parameters in a representative population-based sample of elderly psychotic patients.

We found that 73% of late-onset patients were living alone at time of first hospital contact, while 40% had no contact with any family member. Over half of the cases were described as reclusive, isolatory and "paranoid" for many years preceding illness onset. A third of patients were reported to have impaired hearing, and 20% were visually impaired, with 12% having impairment in both modalities. There was no statistically significant association between modality of sensory impairment and modality of hallucination. However, patients with premorbid paranoid personality traits were significantly less likely than those without such traits to have visual impairment (RR = 0.22; 95% CI = 0.05–0.92); there was a trend towards a similar inverse relationship with hearing impairment (RR = 0.35; 95% CI = 0.11–1.16).

DISCUSSION

Rates of late-onset schizophrenia

There have been very few community-based studies of late-onset schizophrenia. Post (1966) has outlined the difficulties inherent in such studies, pointing to the fact that Kay, Beamish, and Roth (1964), in a community study, identified no patients fulfilling Roth's (1955) criteria for late paraphrenia among 309 persons over 65 years of age in Newcastle, while it was later found that at least 8 patients from that population had been hospitalised or institutionalised with late paraphrenia. In community surveys, Parsons (1964) found a prevalence of late paraphrenia of 1.7% of over-65s in a Welsh town, and Williamson et al. (1964) 1% in a Scottish borough. Christenson and Blazer (1984) found that 4% of 997 elderly persons exhibited symptoms of pervasive persecutory delusions.

Studies of treated rates of late-onset schizophrenia have been reviewed by Harris & Jeste (1988), who noted a marked inconsistency in the reported findings, due, inter alia, to differing case-finding methodology, and a failure to employ standardised diagnostic criteria. On the basis of those eight studies which reported the occurrence of late-onset schizo-phrenia among schizophrenia patients of varying ages, Harris and Jeste estimated (weighted means based on sample size) that around 23% of schizophrenic patients could be considered to have a late-onset of illness (generally onset > 40 years); the range was 15.4% to 32.0%. The mean proportion of late-onset schizophrenics amongst populations of elderly patients with schizophrenia was 31%.

Ten of the studies reviewed by Harris and Jeste reported on differences in the proportion of schizophrenics with age at onset before and after age 60 years. The weighted means showed that around 14% of late-onset (usually > 40 years) schizophrenia patients first manifest the illness after

60. Six of the studies gave a further breakdown of age at onset. Amongst the late-onset patients (onset > 40), a mean of 12.3% had an onset after the age of 60, equivalent to around 3% of all patients with schizophrenia.

In the current study, 16% of the patients had an onset of illness over the age of 60. These figures are rather higher than the proportions estimated by Harris and Jeste (1988), and probably reflect the fact that many earlier studies were prejudiced by the belief that schizophrenia does not manifest for the first time in late life. Also, we included all contacts with the psychiatric services, irrespective of admission, whilst most previous studies have included only those patients actually admitted to hospital; patients with a late onset of illness might well be less likely to require admission to hospital, given their generally better social functioning, the encapsulation of their delusions, and the relative preservation of personality.

In terms of diagnostic criteria fulfilled, only 37% of the very early cases fulfilled DSM-III-R criteria for schizophrenia, whilst over half of the over-60s met the criteria. Few other studies have reported on how many patients with late-onset psychosis fulfil operationalised definitions for schizophrenia, but Rabins, Paulker, and Thomas (1984) found that 21 of 35 (60%) of their group of patients with onset after 44 years met DSM-III criteria for schizophrenia after the age-at-onset stipulation was removed. Thus, the manifestation of stringently defined schizophrenia is by no means confined to younger ages: in the current sample, the annual rate for non-affective functional psychoses in patients over 60 was 13.4 per 100,000, and for DSM-III-R schizophrenia, 7.5 per 100,000; again, low numbers make the confidence limits wide.

Gender

Gender differences in late-onset schizophrenia have been widely reported, with a marked excess of females being seen in almost all pertinent studies, with the male:female ratio in over 60s ranging from 3:1 (Roth, 1955) to 45:2 (Herbert & Jacobsen, 1967). Many of these studies, however, were confined to hospitalised patients, with inherent biases towards more severely affected individuals.

However, the results from this catchment area-based sample of all contacts with the psychiatric services (not only admissions) confirm the female preponderance in later-onset schizophrenia, and particularly in those patients with a very late-onset form of illness. Gender differences in schizophrenia and related disorders have been addressed in Chapters 4 and 5. As stated there, the marked female preponderance in very late-onset cases is difficult to reconcile with the notion that oestrogens "protect" women from manifesting schizophrenia in the reproductive years. An alternative explanation may lie in the literature on differential effects of ageing on male and female brains (see Murphy et al., 1996).

Phenomenology

There have been numerous descriptions of phenomenology in those patients with a very late onset of illness (> 60 years). Castle and Howard (1992), in reviewing such studies, concluded that, in general, such patients were more likely than their early onset counterparts to exhibit paranoid delusions, expressly in the form of highly systematised belief systems; and to have hallucinations in multiple sensory modalities, whilst being generally less likely to show formal thought disorder and "negative" symptoms. There have been few comparative studies of early- and late-onset cases of schizophrenia. Pearlson et al. (1989) conducted a case review and found that, compared to their early-onset counterparts, schizophrenics with an onset of illness after the age of 44 were more likely to be deluded and to experience hallucinations; in contrast, they were much less likely to exhibit formal thought disorder or affective blunting. However, these workers did not specifically address the very late-onset group.

We are aware of no previous large epidemiologically based study comparing phenomenology in late- and early-onset patients, using systematic delineation of symptoms. Of course, retrospective reviews of case records could be biased by differential reporting of symptoms, but this would only be of concern in a comparison study should there be systematic bias in reporting of symptoms in early- and late-onset cases; the fact that some symptoms were found to be more common in the former, and some in the latter groups, suggests this was not the case.

Premorbid functioning and aetiological parameters

Previous investigators (e.g. Kay & Roth, 1961; Post, 1966) have noted that many very late-onset schizophrenia patients have been rather socially isolated throughout their lives, often being described as "odd" or even "paranoid"; some would fulfil criteria for a paranoid personality disorder. The contribution of such personality traits to the later manifestation of psychosis is complex, but clearly reflects a propensity to deal with the world in a certain way, making the manifestation of florid psychosis in the setting of other stressors understandable.

In contrast to their social maladjustment, individuals with a very late-onset of psychosis are reportedly well adjusted in terms of occupational functioning. This puts them apart from their early-onset counterparts, and reinforces our belief, articulated in Chapters 4 and 5, that very early-onset schizophrenia is a pernicious form of the illness which is particularly likely to follow on from premorbid dysfunction.

Aetiological parameters have been underinvestigated in patients with very late-onset "functional" psychoses. Castle and Howard (1992) reviewed published studies of familial aggregation in such illnesses. Many such studies are methodologically problematic, including lack of stringent definition of illness, and lack of control groups. However, the broad conclusion was that very late-onset cases show lower familial loading than those with an early-onset illness, a conclusion consonant with the data reported here. The nature of this case record review study makes the data on familial aggregation suboptimal, although we do not suspect systematic reporting bias.

In line with prediction, obstetric complications and developmental delay were more commonly reported in patients with a very early-onset illness, in line with the view that such patients have a form of illness consequent upon neurodevelopmental deviance (see Murray et al., 1992). The high rates of sensory impairment in the very late-onset group is also in keeping with the literature (reviewed by Castle & Howard, 1992). Of interest is the inverse correlation between premorbid dysfunction and sensory impairment in our sample, suggesting that these are relatively independent predisposing factors rather than cumulative ones (see Castle et al., 1997).

CONCLUSION

We report here the epidemiology of late-onset schizophrenia in a case register sample, and include a systematic analysis of differences between cases with an early and late onset of illness. The findings reinforce the previous reports of a significant minority of patients with a late and very late onset of a schizophrenia-like illness, and delineate differences between such cases and their early-onset counterparts in terms of premorbid functioning and phenomenology; a number of putative aetiological factors were also differentially distributed between these groups. In sum, these findings suggest that it is premature to consider early- and late-onset schizophrenics homogeneous, and there are implications for the understanding of the aetiology of this group of conditions.

CHAPTER SEVEN

Crime and schizophrenia in Camberwell

Recent changes in the care of those with severe mental illness have increased interest in this area, allied to the intense publicity accorded a series of homicides committed in the UK by individuals with a mental disorder. Whether or not such crimes are linked either to mental illness per se, or to recent changes in the care of the mentally ill, remains disputed. Nevertheless, few can doubt that these problems have had an impact, in the UK at least, on recent government policy and legislation on the care of the mentally ill.

Although there is a large literature on the relationship between crime and mental disorder, conclusions conflict and two opposing schools of thought exist on the relationship between crime, violence, and psychosis. One, which Wessely and Taylor (1991) labelled the "criminological" position, is that there is no special association between criminality and mental illness, and that crime committed by the mentally ill is determined by the same factors as in the rest of the population. Support for this view comes from studies showing that criminal behaviour among the mentally ill is associated with the familiar variables, most particularly a history of criminality before the onset of illness.

The alternative argument, which Wessely & Taylor (1991) called the "psychiatric position", is that criminal behaviour (in particular, violence) and serious mental illness coexist more than can be explained by chance, and the nature of this relationship suggests that in a proportion of cases this may have aetiological significance. Advocates of this view cite a series of studies showing an increased rate of offending amongst discharged schizophrenia patients, compared to non-psychiatric controls; to studies of high rates of psychosis in prisoners on remand in UK jails; and to a considerable literature documenting violent behaviour by psychiatric patients both before and during hospital admission.

Taking a typical example, in a sample restricted to first episodes of schizophrenia, Johnstone, Crow, Johnson, and Macmillan (1986) found that 94 patients (37%) had been violent in the previous month, and 22% had had police contact (MacMillan & Johnson, 1987). On closer analysis, 52 cases (20%) were reported to have behaved in a potentially life threatening manner (Humphreys, Johnstone, MacMillan, & Taylor, 1992). Another informative study of the mental health of offenders was carried out in Brixton Prison, a large remand prison, where the prevalence of psychoses in general, and of schizophrenia in particular, was substantially elevated (Taylor, 1985; Taylor & Gunn, 1984).

Much of the seemingly irreconcilable differences in the literature on crime and psychosis can be explained by methodological differences in, and weaknesses of, the various studies. For example, with the exception of homicide, criminal statistics are not an accurate reflection of criminal offending. As far back as 1941 it was pointed out that "the police, as well as the prosecutor, act more efficiently in the case of serious crimes than otherwise" (Inghe, 1941). The clear up rate depends on the severity of the crime; the chances of identification of the perpetrator also increases with the severity. Fortunately for epidemiological studies such as the one we report here, however, the correlation between official crime and true offending behaviour, as measured by self-report, is reasonably strong, especially for more serious offences (Farrington, 1973; Huizinga & Elliot, 1986). There is a strong association between official measures of criminal behaviour and measures of violent behaviour that did not result in arrest (Link, Andrews, & Cullen, 1992), leading Farrington to state that "conclusions about characteristics of offenders based on convictions were generally similar to conclusions based upon self-reports of offending."

Other biases are common. For example, the presence of mental illness often reduces the likelihood of criminal prosecution and conviction. When a US attorney rated the records of patients admitted to a state mental hospital, he concluded that 71% of patients had committed illegal acts before admission. In the Northwick Park study (Johnstone, Leary, Frith, & Owens, 1991), 38 patients had had contact with the police before admission, but had not been charged. On the other hand, being mentally ill means the perpetrator is more likely to be detected during the commission of the crime (Robertson,1988).

Another factor is that, after detection, mental illness may decrease the probability of the individual being labelled a criminal, and people who are viewed by the police or the courts as mentally ill may be less likely to be prosecuted (Klassen & O'Connor, 1988; Mackay & Wight, 1984). That the police are reluctant to arrest and prosecute, the courts to convict, and the prisons to house, the mentally abnormal offender is clearly desirable on humanitarian grounds, but has implications for the accuracy of criminological data.

Some differences in studies can be attributed to selection bias. For example, in the numerous studies of the outcome of patients discharged from US state mental hospitals, like is not being compared to like. Other problems are related to confounding. For example, there is little doubt of the association between alcohol and crime. Hence the finding that in one oft-quoted study of a mainly schizophrenic cohort, 66% of participants had an alcohol problem (Giovannoni & Gurel, 1967).

THE CURRENT STUDY

A powerful way of studying the relationship between crime and psychosis is to use a cohort design, sometimes called in this context a "criminal careers" approach. The Camberwell Register sample gave us the opportunity to carry out such a study using an incident cohort of those with schizophrenia, compared to community controls matched for age, gender, period, and the presence of any mental disorder. The full results of the study are contained in Wessely (1994), and a precis in Wessely, Castle, Douglas, and Taylor (1994).

A variety of factors influence offending, each of which are influenced by time. First, it is well known that age is strongly related to criminal activity. Second, external influences, such as a change in the method of recording crime, a period of high unemployment, wartime and so on, exert influences on all age groups ("period effects"). Third, some factors are restricted to one birth group ("cohort effects"). One way of addressing these issues is by so-called "age–period–cohort" models. However, the age–period–cohort model is difficult to comprehend, and can only be appreciated statistically. The current study was designed to avoid the necessity of using such complex models, substituting instead more conventional methods of cohort analysis.

For this study, the cohort consists of individuals identified during their first episode of psychosis, and then followed up over time to determine the nature and rate of criminal convictions. The cases are therefore the same cases of schizophrenia and related disorders as in the previous chapters (see Chapters 2 and 3 for details of patient selection, diagnostic breakdown, etc.).

The problem of age and period effects was overcome by recruiting a control cohort, which would experience the same changes of age, period, and cohort as the study cohort. For each case a control was recruited, matched for age, gender, and period. Each case–control pair therefore experienced the same influences of age and period, and any observed differences between cohorts would not be due to these confounding factors.

As the aim of the study was to consider the influence of schizophrenia on offending, the control cohort was chosen to resemble the study cohort in as many ways as practicable. We have already pointed out that little purpose would be served by further comparisons of selected groups of mentally abnormal offenders with so-called "normal" groups. Thus, controls were the next person on the Camberwell Cumulative Psychiatric Case Register of appropriate age and sex, but not suffering from schizophrenia or a related disorder.

Time at risk

Time at risk is a crucial concept in any study of schizophrenia and crime. In general, people are not able to acquire a criminal record whilst either in prison, or in hospital. There are exceptions to this, since theoretically they can be prosecuted for offences which take place either in prison or hospital, but in practice admission to an institution, either a prison or a hospital, means the individual is at considerably reduced risk of acquiring a criminal record. Because admission to hospital is not random, failure to control for this would add a substantial bias to any study comparing offending rates of mentally ill persons, contrasted to those without a mental illness. To date no study has adequately addressed this issue. Although the current study does not use a "normal" control sample, time at risk is likely to differ between cases with psychosis, and controls with other mental illnesses, since the former are more likely to spend prolonged periods in hospital.

To take account of such factors, time at risk for acquiring a criminal record was calculated for each person in the study. Since 1964, the start of this study, the minimum age for criminal responsibility has been 10. Therefore, they could not be at risk of acquiring a conviction before that age, and therefore do not contribute person years until age 10. No adjustment needs to be made for those entering the United Kingdom from elsewhere before the age of 10. However, adjustment was made for the following:

1. Age at entry to United Kingdom (if over 10)
2. Time in prison.
3. Time in hospital.
4. Date of any immigration or emigration.
5. Date of death.

Details of all participants for whom the case records did not clearly indicate a date of death, or who were not in contact with the local mental health services at the termination of the study, were sent to the Office of Population Censuses and Surveys. Dates were obtained of all "exit events": death, emigration, or entering a long-stay hospital (defined as a stay of longer than two years). Time in hospital was obtained from local hospital case records, supplemented by the computerised or non-computerised administrative records maintained at all the local hospitals. The Camberwell Case Register also contained dates of all hospital admissions, which were used for all those with missing or inadequate records, or with long gaps in the case records. This method ensured that virtually all admissions of cases and controls to catchment area hospitals were recorded. Requests for information from other hospitals, were also followed up; even when complete records were not available, we could obtain dates of admissions. A check was also made on the Special Hospital Case Register for any cases admitted to one of the Special Hospitals in England and Wales. For those no longer in contact, or whose case records had been destroyed, general practitioners were traced via OPCS and asked for simple information including dates of admission.

Criminal record data

Criminal record data were requested on the entire sample, including those with missing case records. These data were provided by the Criminal Records Office (CRO). A summary statistic giving the total number of offences, further divided into those that occurred before the onset of illness, and those either simultaneous with, or after, illness onset, was calculated from the CRO records and case records for each participant. Offence categories were then divided as follows:

1. Theft (burglary; theft; stealing; receiving stolen property; conspiracy to rob; larceny; taking and driving away motor vehicle; obtaining property by deception).
2. Criminal damage (criminal damage; breach of the peace; using offensive language; malicious damage; possessing offensive weapon; suspected person).
3. Assault and violence (actual and grievous bodily harm; attempted homicide; manslaughter; arson; malicious wounding; assault).
4. Sexual offences (indecency; exposing; indecent assault; incest; prostitution; unlawful sexual intercourse).
5. Drug and alcohol offences (drunk and disorderly; driving with excess alcohol; possessing illegal substances; using forged prescription to obtain drugs).

6. A residual category was created for various offences that occurred rarely (often with only one example) and could not be easily classified elsewhere. These included possessing firearms without a certificate; perjury; begging; insurance offences; running a disorderly house; and dangerous driving.

An analysis based solely on offences would overestimate the number of separate offending events, since one event could lead to several convictions. As Farrington (1990) has pointed out, a burglar arrested for a single event could face charges of "going equipped" as well as burglary. For that reason, we employed Farrington's method of rating separately only offences committed on different days. If two or more offences occurred on the same day, only the most serious was rated.

The Criminal Records Office may not record every conviction obtained. Some convictions simply never get recorded due to administrative failures. There is some evidence that these false negatives increase with the distance from London (Steer, 1973; West & Farrington, 1973). Steer (1973) estimated that about 10% of indictable offences are not recorded at the CRO. Fortunately, the current study was based in London, suggesting a lower rate of unrecorded offence.

All case records were routinely assessed for evidence of a criminal history, as part of a reliability check, and also to determine the accuracy of forensic history-taking by psychiatrists (see Wessely & Castle, 1992). Twenty-one case records contained details of convictions that were not recorded on the CRO. There are a number of explanations for these apparent false–positive case records. First, records are removed ("cleaned") from the CRO when the individual dies. However, the CRO are not informed by the Office of Population Census and Surveys (OPCS) of death, which suggests that cleaning must be relatively ineffective. In this study, 12 (7%) of those individuals recorded at OPCS as dead, still had an entry in the CRO.

Records are routinely cleaned after 20 years if no further offending has taken place. However, there are a number of exceptions to this, specifically if the offence led to imprisonment, if the person has a mental history (although it is not clear how this is ascertained), or if the conviction involved drugs or violence, or was a sexual offence. Contacts with the Criminal Record Office also reveal a shortage of funds to carry out this policy. It seems that such cleaning has had little, if any, effect on this cohort.

A number of offences are not routinely included in individual criminal record data. Motoring offences, prostitution, licence offences and, more recently, cannabis smoking are all offences, but are not routinely measured. Similarly, although the number of cautions administered are recorded, they are not listed by individual. All such data would therefore be absent from both cases and controls.

Mentally ill offenders found guilty may receive a Section 37 Order. On making such an order the magistrate has the power to quash any conviction, which will thus not be recorded at the CRO. This power is not available in the Crown Court, and thus Section 37/41 (Restriction Orders) do appear on the CRO records.

Adjustment was therefore made for the above exceptions. Only 13 case records contained convictions which should have appeared in the CRO records. This represents only 5% of the convictions obtained from the CRO, and suggests that the CRO was an accurate source of outcome data.

One female case with over 100 convictions for prostitution would have resulted in substantial distortions in the analysis, and was treated as an outlier. She was arbitrarily coded as having one pre- and one post- illness offence.

Analysis

This study allowed two different analytical approaches to be taken. The first is a comparison of two cohorts, one containing those with schizophrenia, the other controls without schizophrenia. Both cases and controls are followed up over a period, during which time they are able to acquire any number of criminal convictions. Knowing both the time at risk and the number of offences, the true rates of offending can be calculated for both cases and controls. These rates can then be compared, the resulting measure being a rate ratio.

The design permits a second type of analysis. Each participant has the potential risk of obtaining a conviction during the study period. It is possible to calculate the strength of the association between a number of variables (which could include schizophrenia, but also such social variables as class, employment, and so on) and the risk of acquiring any lifetime conviction, or the risk of acquiring a conviction after the onset of schizophrenia. Survival analysis ascertains not only who obtains a conviction, but also the length of time it takes them to do so. Survival analysis allows adjustment for certain confounders, such as substance misuse, gender, social class, and others.

Rates of conviction

Unadjusted rate ratios for specific offences are shown in Table 7.1a and b for all diagnoses, and for DSM-III–R diagnoses, respectively. Considering all diagnostic groups, males showed an excess of violent offending, whilst females showed an excess of both assault and of theft. In those patients with DSM-III–R defined schizophrenia, theft was again significantly more

TABLE 7.1a
Rate Ratios For Specific Offences In Cases Versus Controls: All ICD-9 Diagnoses

	Males		Females	
Offence	Rate ratio (95% CI)	P-value	Rate ratio (95% CI)	P-value
All	1.0 (0.9–1.2)	.27	3.3 (2.3–4.7)	<.0001
Assault and serious violence	2.1 (1.5–2.9)	<.001	3.1 (1.3–7.4)	.005
Theft	0.9 (0.8–1.0)	.04	3.1 (2.0–4.7)	<.0001
Criminal damage	1.2 (0.9–1.6)	.09	2.5 (0.8–8.0)	.10
Alcohol and drug-related	0.9 (0.6–1.3)	.19	—	—
Sexual	0.8 (0.4–1.6)	.20	6.6 (0.8–54.7)	.05

(From Wessely et al., 1994. Reprinted with the permission of Cambridge University Press.)

TABLE 7.1b
Rate Ratios For Specific Offences In Cases Versus Controls: DSM-III–R
Schizophrenia Only

	Males		Females	
Offence	Rate ratio (95% CI)	P-value	Rate ratio (95% CI)	P-value
All	1.4 (1.2–1.5)	<.001	4.1 (1.7–10.0)	<.001
Assault and serious violence	3.1 (1.8–5.5)	.01	—	—
Theft	0.9 (0.7–1.2)	.25	3.8 (1.3–11.5)	<.001
Criminal damage	2.0 (1.2–3.2)	.003	2.0 (0.4–11.1)	.33
Alcohol and drug-related	1.3 (0.7–2.4)	.29	—	—
Sexual	0.5 (0.2–1.5)	.07	—	—

(From Wessely et al., 1994. Reprinted with the permission of Cambridge University Press.)

common amongst affected females, whilst assault and criminal damage were characteristics associated with schizophrenic males.

The rate ratios presented in Table 7.1a and b are unadjusted, although the sampling strategy means that there is no confounding effect of time period or age, confirmed by negative tests for heterogeneity. The influence of gender, class, and ethnicity is complicated. In the women there was no evidence of heterogeneity between the strata (class, ethnicity), and thus adjustment for both class and ethnicity could be made using Poisson regression available on the EGRET statistical package. The rate ratio for effect of schizophrenia on offending in women was 2.1 (95% CI = 1.4–3.1) adjusted for social class and ethnicity.

However, a more complex picture emerged in the men. There was evidence for heterogeneity by ethnic group, but not class. The rate ratio for the effect of schizophrenia in African-Caribbeans, adjusted for class, was 3.4 (95% CI = 1.9–6.3), but in the other ethnic groups combined (nearly all Caucasians) it was 0.6 (95% CI = 0.5–0.7). Thus, schizophrenia considerably increased the risk of offending in African-Caribbean men, but not other groups. The overall rate ratio for the effect of schizophrenia, which was close to unity, in fact comprises two opposing effects.

Age at first conviction

Cases began their criminal career significantly later than controls (controls 21.7 years; 95% CI = 20.0–23.5; cases 24.6 years 95% CI = 22.8–26.3; $t = -2.24$, 248 df, $P = .03$). Turning to within-group differences, the close relationship between age at onset, age at first offence, and diagnosis noted elsewhere (Coid, 1983) was confirmed. Using DSM-III criteria (which have an age cut-off for schizophrenia at 44 years), the mean age at onset versus mean age at first conviction for the affective diagnoses was 30.8 versus 28.1; that for schizophrenia was 25.4 (age at onset) versus 23.5 (age at first conviction).

Predictors of first conviction

Table 7.2a, b, c shows unadjusted odds ratios for a range of parameters considered in attempting to delineate those factors predictive of a first criminal conviction. It will be noted that some factors, notably being male, abusing illicit substances, and having an early onset of illness, were associated with criminal conviction for both cases and controls. In contrast, African-Caribbean ethnicity and being single were predictors only for schizophrenia patients.

Using Cox's Proportional Hazards modelling, it was possible to adjust for confounding factors, and to determine independent effects associated with a first criminal conviction. Thus, the factors were: being of African-Caribbean ethnicity (hazard ratio (HR) = 2.3; 95% CI = 1.6–3.2); being male (HR = 3.3; 95% CI = 2.5–4.0); and using illicit substances (HR = 2.5; 95% CI = 1.7–3.5). In terms of illness, there were positive independent associations between first criminal conviction and having schizophrenia (HR = 1.4; 95% CI = 1.0–2.0). Early illness onset also had a significant effect (HR = 1.05; 95% CI = 1.04–1.07).

In patients with schizophrenia, a number of parameters predicted first conviction, notably ethnicity, male sex, substance use, early illness onset, and poor premorbid adjustment (see Table 7.3). In this group, social class, marital status, and employment status did not predict criminality.

TABLE 7.2a
Factors Contributing To First Criminal Offence: Unadjusted (Crude) Odds Ratio:
(Dichotomous Data)

	Cases: (ICD-9 schizophrenia: n=538)			Controls (other mental disorders: n=538)		
	Odds ratio	95% CI	P-value	Odds ratio	95% CI	P-value
DSM-III-R Schiz. spectrum[1]	1.5	1.0–2.2	.05	—	—	—
DSM-III-R Schiz.[2]	1.3	0.9–2.0	.13	—	—	—
Female	0.2	0.1–0.3	<.001	0.2	0.1–0.4	<.001
Job	0.6	0.4–0.9	.02	—	—	—
Unemp.	1.7	1.1–2.6	.053	—	—	—
Ethnicity[3]	2.6	1.7–4.0	<.001	1.6	0.7–3.4	.23
Premorbid work adjustment	2.5	1.6–3.8	<.001	—	—	—
Premorbid social adjustment	2.1	1.4–3.2	<.001	—	—	—
Subst. Abuse[4]	4.9	2.8–8.4	<.001	3.8	2.3–6.2	<.001
Married[5]	0.5	0.3–0.8	<.001	0.7	0.4–1.1	.21

[1] Versus ICD-9 psychoses.
[2] Versus ICD-9 psychoses.
[3] Ethnicity compares all Afro-Caribbeans with all other groups. It is by ethnicity, and not place of birth.
[4] Drugs and alcohol indicate any harmful use.
[5] Being married or living as married are coded together.
(From Wessely et al., 1994. Reprinted with the permission of Cambridge University Press.)

Post-illness conviction

To model post-illness convictions, a similar plan of analysis, moving from crude odds ratios to an adjusted regression model, was used with some modifications. When offence and illness onset appeared to be simultaneous, an arbitrary figure of one month was used for time to post-illness conviction, in order to permit the application of survival analysis.

Unadjusted odds ratios were obtained to determine the influence of key predictor variables on post-illness conviction (Table 7.4a and b). Cox's Proportional Hazard modelling was again used to determine the fully adjusted associations of post-illness conviction across the cohort. As before, an unadjusted analysis was carried out in the cases and controls separately (Table 7.5), and a fully adjusted model developed for the cases alone (Table 7.6).

TABLE 7.2b
Factors Contributing To First Criminal Offence: Unadjusted (Crude) Odds Ratio:
(Polychotomous Data)

	Cases: (ICD-9 schizophrenia)			Controls (other mental disorders)		
	Odds ratio	95% CI	P-value	Odds ratio	95% CI	P-value
Social Class III	1.7	0.9–3.3	.07	1.6	0.6–4.0	.24
Social Class IV & V	1.8	0.9–3.4	.06[1]	1.3	0.6–3.2	.50[2]
Period 1970–74	0.9	0.5–1.6	.40	1.2	0.6–2.4	.65
1975–1979	1.1	0.6–2.0	.47	1.6	0.8–3.1	.16
1980–1984	1.5	0.9–2.7	.07[3]	1.7	0.8–3.3	.12[4]

[1] Test for trend; $P=.114$.
[2] Test for trend: $P=.828$.
[3] Test for trend: $P=.04$.
[4] Test for trend; $P=.078$.
(From Wessely et al., 1994. Reprinted with the permission of Cambridge University Press.)

TABLE 7.2c
Unadjusted (Crude) Odds Ratios: Continuous Data (Cox's Proportional Hazard Model)

	Cases			Controls		
	Hazard ratio	95% CI	P-value	Hazard ratio	95% CI	P-value
Age of onset of illness	.95	0.93–0.96	<.001	.93	0.91–0.95	<.001

Broadly defined schizophrenia was significantly associated with obtaining a criminal conviction after the onset of illness, with almost a twofold increase in risk (odds ratio (OR)=1.8; 95% CI=1.3–2.6). A very similar range of factors were all significantly associated with criminality after the onset of illness (Table 7.4). Age of onset of illness remained associated (cases, HR=0.94; 95% CI=0.92–0.96), but not age at first offence. Looking at cases and controls together in the fully adjusted model (Table 7.4), previous conviction, gender, ethnicity, substance abuse, and age of onset of illness continued to be significant, but not for clinically defined schizophrenia. However, in the cases alone (Table 7.5), there is a weak trend for an increased risk for DSM-III-R schizophrenia over broadly defined schizophrenia (Table 7.6).

TABLE 7.3
Independent Risk Factors Contributing To First Conviction In Patients With Clinically
Defined Schizophrenia; Adjusted Model: Cases only: Cox's Proportional Hazards;
n=538

Term	Coefficient	Hazard ratio	95% CI	P-value
Ethnicity	.7661	2.2	1.5–3.1	< .001
Being female	−1.112	0.3	0.2–0.5	< .001
Substance abuse	.6831	2.0	1.2–3.4	.01
Age onset of illness	−.0464	0.95	0.94–0.98	< .001
Poor premorbid adjustment	.4509	1.6	1.0–2.5	.07
Schizophrenia (DSM-III–R)	.2383	1.3	0.9–1.8	.19
Social class	.1425	1.2	0.9–1.5	.27
Being married	.2400	1.3	0.8–2.0	.29
Job	−.2315	0.8	0.5–1.2	.31
Unemployed	−.1027	0.9	0.6–1.4	.63

(From Wessely et al., 1994. Reprinted with the permission of Cambridge University Press.)

DISCUSSION

In this study, we tested the hypothesis that schizophrenia is associated with an increased risk of criminal conviction compared to other mental disorders (controls). The controls were a random sample of patients with non-psychotic mental disorders, recorded on the Camberwell Case

TABLE 7.4a
Predictors Of First Post-Illness Conviction In ICD-9 Schizophrenia Versus Other
Mental Disorders; Crude (Unadjusted) Odds Ratios: Dichotomous Data

	Cases: (ICD-9 schizophrenia)			Controls (other mental disorders)		
	Odds ratio	95% CI	P-value	Odds ratio	95% CI	P-value
DSM-III–R schiz. spectrum	1.5	1.0–2.4	.06	—	—	—
DSM-III–R schiz.	1.6	1.0–2.5	.04	—	—	—
Being female	0.2	0.1–0.4	< .001	0.2	0.1–0.4	< .001
Job	0.7	0.4–1.1	.12	—	—	—
Unemp.	2.0	1.2–3.2	.004	—	—	—
Prev. crim. rec.	8.2	4.9–13.9	< .001	23.1	12.6–44.6	< .001
Ethnicity	3.6	3.3–5.7	< .001	2.1	0.9–4.8	.07
Substance abuse	4.2	2.4–7.4	< .001	5.3	2.5–11.8	< .001
Married	0.4	0.2–0.6	< .001	0.7	0.4–1.3	.24

(From Wessely et al., 1994. Reprinted with the permission of Cambridge University Press.)

TABLE 7.4b
Unadjusted (Crude) Odds Ratio For Post-Illness Offending (Polychotomous Data)

	Cases: (ICD-9 schizophrenia)			Controls (other mental disorders)		
	Odds ratio	95% CI	P-value	Odds ratio	95% CI	P-value
Social Class III	1.4	0.7–3.0	.27	0.9	0.3–2.6	.83
Social Class IV & V	1.6	0.8–3.3	.17[1]	1.3	0.5–3.4	.64[2]
Period 1970–74	1.0	0.5–1.9	.93	1.3	0.6–2.9	.48
1975–1979	1.2	0.7–2.4	.40	1.1	0.5–2.4	.84
1980–1984	1.5	0.8–2.7	.24[3]	1.2	0.5–2.7	.62[4]

[1] Test for trend; $P = .21$.
[2] Test for trend; $P = .43$.
[3] Test for trend: $P = .16$.
[4] Test for trend; $P = .77$.
(From Wessely et al., 1994. Reprinted with the permission of Cambridge University Press.)

Register. They thus included substantial numbers of individuals, especially in the men, with diagnoses known to be associated with offending, such as substance abuse and personality disorder. The study therefore tests the hypothesis that schizophrenia per se, rather than all forms of mental illness, is associated with an increased risk of criminality.

The main limitation of the study is that it consists solely of detected criminality, and is thus subject to the many biases that intervene between offending and criminal conviction, as discussed in the introduction to this chapter. The choice of controls reduces some of these biases, such as the stigma of mental disorder and the ease of detection of mentally abnormal offenders, but certainly does not eliminate it. We thus report a study of detected criminality, rather than offending behaviour in general.

TABLE 7.5
Adjusted Model: Post-Illness First Conviction: Cases And Controls
Combined (n=1076): Cox's Proportional Hazards

Term	Hazard ratio	95% CI	P-value
Previous conviction	3.9	2.71–5.63	< .001
Ethnicity	2.3	1.56–3.30	< .001
Being female	0.4	0.24–0.60	< .001
Substance abuse	1.6	0.99–2.58	.055
Age onset of illness	0.95	0.93–0.97	< .001
Schizophrenia (ICD-9)	1.4	0.86–2.13	.185

(From Wessely et al., 1994. Reprinted with the permission of Cambridge University Press.)

TABLE 7.6
Independent Predictors of Post-Illness First Conviction in ICD-9 Schizophrenia
(*n*=538): Cox's Proportional Hazards Model: Fully Adjusted

Variable	Coeff.	SE	Hazard ratio	95% CI	P-value
Prev. conviction	1.016	.231	2.8	1.9–4.5	< .001
Ethnicity	0.8074	.217	2.2	1.5–3.2	< .001
Substance abuse	0.5870	.233	1.8	1.2–2.7	.012
DSM-III-R schiz.	0.3641	.214	1.4	0.9–2.1	.09
Age of onset of illness	−0.5569	.140	0.95	0.93–0.97	< .001
Being female	−0.8286	.284	0.4	0.3–0.7	.004

(Reprinted with the permission of Cambridge University Press.)

On the other hand, the study has important advantages. Participants were incident cases. The use of the Camberwell Case Register to identify cases, rather than relying on hospital discharges as have most other studies, is an important issue, since violent behaviour is a frequent reason for admission to hospital, as we have shown in this data set (see Chapter 3), and thus is a potentially important confounder of any observed relationship between crime and mental disorder in which subjects are identified at hospital discharge (Marzuk, 1996).

We have shown that men with schizophrenia do not have an overall increased risk of criminality compared to men with other mental disorders. This risk increases with more stringent definitions of schizophrenia, but is never substantial. However, the risk of being convicted for a violent offence is at least twice that of men with other non-psychotic mental disorders. Women with schizophrenia have an overall increased risk of acquiring any conviction.

Looking at the age of first conviction (Fig. 7.1), cases and controls did not differ in early years, but deviated more with increasing age. The data on the controls do not differ from national data acquired in the middle of the study period (Farrington, 1981). This is consistent with several studies that have found a later mean age of first conviction in very selected groups of mentally disordered offenders compared to "normal" offenders.

Comparison with other studies

Our results are consistent with the modern generation of studies of crime and mental illness. They join a series of six contemporary studies all of which report an association between crime and schizophrenia.

Two of these are true community studies. In the first, Swanson, Holzer, Ganju, and Jono (1990) performed a secondary analysis of the ECA data set, using the four questions included for the diagnosis of antisocial personality disorder. They found that all psychiatric diagnoses, including

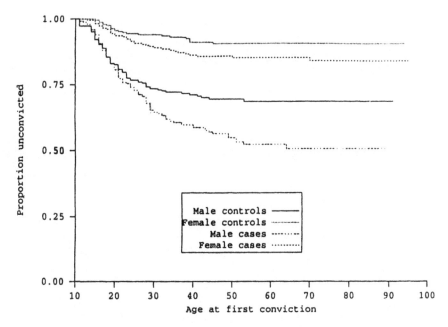

FIG. 7.1. Time to first conviction. (Reprinted with the permission of Cambridge University Press.)

schizophrenia, were associated with a substantially increased risk of recalling violent behaviours, even after controlling for important confounders such as age, gender, and social class.

The second study (Link et al., 1992) compared samples of psychiatric patients and community residents drawn from the same deprived area of New York City. Not only were official arrest records obtained, but also all participants were interviewed concerning self-reported arrests, and questioned about antisocial behaviours, including hitting others, fighting, using weapons, and "hurting someone badly in a fight". The Psychiatric Epidemiology Research Interview (PERI) was used to obtain information about current psychotic symptoms, although not diagnoses. As in the Swanson et al. (1990) study, the patient groups had higher rates of nearly all the variables associated with criminality and/or antisocial behaviour, including arrest rates (especially for violent offences), and all the self-reported indices of antisocial behaviour, apart from violent crimes. The association reduced, but remain significant, once adjustment was made for social confounders. However, the associations with antisocial behaviour ceased to be significant when adjustment was made for current psychotic symptomatology. Controlling for current mental state reduced, but did not eliminate, the association with arrest rates.

The three criminal careers studies all come from Scandinavia. Lindqvist and Allebeck (1990) obtained long-term data on the criminal careers of 644 schizophrenia patients identified during their first hospitalisation. The expected rates of offending were determined by indirect standardisation with national statistics, which were then compared to the observed values. The overall relative risk of offending in males was not significantly elevated, in contrast to the value for females. However, when restricted to violent offending there was an approximately fourfold increase in the risk in people with schizophrenia compared to normals, similar to our results.

In the second study, Hodgins (1992) analysed a birth cohort consisting of all persons born in Stockholm in 1953. Outcome data were again obtained from national sources, supplemented by school, military, and social service records. Data on mental health status came from the Stockholm County Register. The risk of all offences in men who also had a mental health contact was increased by 2.5, rising to 4 for violent offences, while women with a mental health contact had 5 times the risk of acquiring a criminal record, and 27 times of acquiring a criminal record for violence.

Hodgins and her colleagues (1996) also published an analysis of a Danish birth cohort, consisting of all persons born between 1944 and 1947. Once again, those discharged from psychiatric institutions with a major mental disorder (covering all the psychoses) had a threefold increase in the risk of acquiring a criminal conviction.

These three Scandinavian cohort studies represent a substantial advance on previous work in this field. However, all contain a bias towards the more seriously ill by excluding those with schizophrenia never admitted to a psychiatric hospital, and were thus not community based, despite the use of a case register. In the current study, we have shown (Chapter 3) that violent behaviour is associated with hospital admission, and hence that hospital admission is an important potential confounder of any association between crime and mental disorder. Furthermore, in neither Swedish study were corrections made for time at risk. No direct check was made upon the diagnoses obtained from the register. Participants who had died or emigrated were excluded. Both studies terminated relatively early; no data was obtained of convictions or outcome after age 30 in two, although the Danish analysis extended to age 43.

Finally, Modestin and Ammann (1996) carried out a study of the subsequent criminal careers of a consecutive sample of male inpatients with schizophrenia, although these were prevalent and not incident cases. The comparison group were community controls, in which some attempt was made to match for confounders such as age, social class, and marital status. As we found, the overall risk of criminal convictions was not increased, but there were specific and substantial increases in the risk of convictions for violent crimes.

Predictors of conviction

Turning to the predictors of acquiring a criminal record, many of our findings confirm what is known from the criminological literature, enhancing the credibility of the methodology employed. Acquiring any criminal record was more likely in the presence of unemployment, lower social class, substance abuse, and African-Caribbean ethnicity. It was less likely if the person was married, working, or female. All of these had stronger effects, both promoting or preventing criminality, than did the presence of psychosis. Once the effect of confounding variables was taken into account, being a case (i.e. clinically defined schizophrenia) continued to increase significantly the risk of conviction, but greater effects remained for gender, ethnicity, substance abuse, and age of onset (itself a proxy for a number of factors, including age). Social class, marital and employment status, and the more restricted categories of schizophrenia, all made modest contributions, but these were no longer significant.

We have confirmed that social variables continue to be the strongest predictors of criminal behaviour in those with mental illness. However, additional risk is also conveyed by psychosis itself. Using the classification outlined in the introduction to this chapter, the results presented here offer some, albeit limited, support, to the "psychiatric" position: schizophrenia does make a contribution to criminal behaviour, especially violent offending.

Substance abuse independently increased the risk of acquiring a criminal record in the cases confirming the association between schizophrenia, substance abuse, and criminality (see Marzuk, 1996). However, the prevalence of substance abuse was low, in keeping with the literature on substance abuse and schizophrenia (Bernadt & Murray, 1986; Schneier & Siris, 1987). Patients with drug-induced psychosis were excluded from the cohort, together with other organic psychoses. We also calculated the population attributable risk, which can be interpreted as the proportion by which convictions would be reduced if substance abuse could be eliminated from the cohort; this was 16.7%.

The presence of schizophrenia also increased the risk of post-illness conviction nearly twofold. Clinically defined schizophrenia continued to exert an effect, as did more restricted categories of schizophrenia. Survival analysis showed that previous conviction, ethnicity, gender, and substance abuse, but not schizophrenia, remained independent predictors of post-illness conviction. The strongest predictor was that of previous conviction, confirming many other studies. Age of onset of illness continued to exert an independent effect, in that for each year that onset of schizophrenia was delayed, the risk of conviction decreased.

The effect of age of onset of illness is complex. Age at onset of illness and age at first conviction were closely correlated, the younger the age of onset, the younger the age at first conviction. Furthermore, the younger the age of onset, the greater the risk of acquiring any conviction. There are a number of competing explanations. First, is it a methodological artifact? The earlier the age of onset, the greater the number of years left to acquire a criminal conviction. However, this is not the explanation, since the effect was for a lifetime criminal record, not just post-illness conviction.

Second, is the link between age at onset and the risk of criminal conviction due to the particular characteristics of early-onset schizophrenia? Age of onset could be associated with previous antisocial behaviour, as it was in this data set. There is some evidence (Castle & Murray, 1991) that early-onset schizophrenia, particularly in men, has a poor prognosis, and is associated with a higher risk of developmental abnormalities—premorbid offending may thus be part of the prodrome of early-onset illness. Although Hodgins (1992) did not measure age of onset, she noted that "the clinical behaviour of subjects who eventually developed major disorders often appeared in early adolescence, well before the mental disorder would have been diagnosed." Poor premorbid work and social adjustment, rated without knowledge of criminal records, was associated with over a twofold increase in the unadjusted risk of acquiring a criminal record. However, the effect of age of onset is not specific for schizophrenia, since it is also found in the controls. Perhaps early presentation with mental disorder is more likely to be associated with behavioural disturbance in several diagnostic categories.

Ethnicity and age at onset

The influence of African-Caribbean ethnicity on convictions rates is of concern. It was expected that ethnicity would be a strong confounder of any association between crime and schizophrenia. We show in Chapters 8 and 9 that African-Caribbeans in this area of London are at considerably greater risk of schizophrenia than those of other ethnic origins. It is also known that African-Caribbeans have higher rates of criminal conviction than other ethnic groups in the UK (Farrington, 1993). This must in part be due to the greater prevalence of poverty, school failure, family breakdown, and unemployment in the African-Caribbean community in the UK (Brown, 1984), since these are known associations with offending (Farrington & West, 1990).

Another confounder might be age of onset of illness. In the same data set we have shown that males with an early age of onset (before age 25) are characterised by a severe form of schizophrenia, with long duration and lack of affective symptomatology. These patients were more likely than their female counterparts to have remained single, to have poor premorbid social and employment records, and to exhibit personality disorder (see Chapters 4 and 5). The current study suggests that it is these young African-Caribbean men with schizophrenia who also show recidivist criminal behaviour, accounting for the interaction between ethnicity, schizophrenia, and rates of conviction noted in the men, but not women. The role of age of illness onset as a confounder, and hence, a possible explanation of the ethnic differences in criminal convictions, appears to be supported by the finding that the mean age at onset for African-Caribbeans was lower than that for UK-born non-African-Caribbeans (males, 28.3 versus 33.7 years; females, 31.2 versus 46.2 years). However, there was no difference when schizophrenia was diagnosed by DSM-III, which has an upper age limit of 44 years.

The identification of a group of young African-Caribbean men with both schizophrenia and criminal recidivism may explain the otherwise puzzling discrepancy between the effect of ethnicity and gender on the rates of offending and the risk of first offence. In females, the rate of conviction in the cases was twice that of the controls, with no interaction effect for ethnicity; in other words, the influence of schizophrenia on convictions was equal in cases and controls, and permitted the calculation of the rate ratio for the effect of schizophrenia on the rate of conviction in women, adjusted for class and ethnicity ($RR = 2.1$). However, this was not the case in men. Here schizophrenia actually decreased the rate of conviction in non African-Caribbeans, but increased it in African-Caribbeans. In these circumstances it was not possible to calculate a rate adjusted for ethnicity, but simply two rates adjusted for class. This is evidence of an interaction between ethnicity, gender, and schizophrenia on the rate of criminal conviction.

No such interaction was found for the risk of first conviction. Schizophrenia continued to increase the risk of conviction, albeit to a small extent, irrespective of ethnicity. There was no significant interaction term for schizophrenia and ethnicity. These differences can be explained by the existence of a group of young African-Caribbean men with higher rates of recidivism. The particular contribution made by these individuals to the overall rates of conviction explains why the interaction was only noted in the rate ratio analyses (which takes into account the total number of offences), and not of those of first or post-illness conviction.

The effect of ethnicity persisted independently of measures of social deprivation, such as unemployment, social class, and substance abuse, as well as age of illness onset. One possible explanation is that these were inadequate controls for social deprivation. Unemployment and lower social class are only proxy measures for various forms of social deprivation, and may well not be adequate measures. The recording of drug abuse was by no means complete.

Another possible explanation for the ethnicity effect lies in the operation of the criminal justice system. Two London surveys (Smith & Gray, 1983; Stevens & Willis, 1979) provided some evidence that black people were at increased risk of arrest by the police, but were unable to distinguish between such competing explanations as age, socioeconomic status, and place of residence. Crow (1987) argued that this increase in arrests and convictions among black people is because they are more likely to be apprehended, charged, and convicted. It has also been shown that black youths are less likely to be cautioned, and more likely to be prosecuted, than Caucasians (Commission for Racial Equality, 1992; Landau, 1981). However, victim surveys show that police bias is not a complete explanation (see Hindelang, 1983; Home Office Statistical Bulletin, 1989).

The general effect of ethnicity on conviction, as seen in cases and controls, could also be due to selection bias. It is possible that African-Caribbeans only come to the attention of mental health services in the context of disturbed behaviour, unlike Caucasians. However, although this is a plausible argument for the control sample, it is unlikely to be relevant to the cases. We have already noted that nearly all individuals with schizophrenia come to the attention of the mental health services, especially in countries with well-developed community services. No evidence has been presented from community studies of substantial numbers of participants with psychosis and no history of contact with mental health services. We have also found no evidence that the diagnosis of schizophrenia in African-Caribbeans is influenced by a history of disturbed behaviour. Despite occasional assertions to the contrary, racial bias in the diagnosis of schizophrenia in the United Kingdom has not been substantiated (Lewis, Croft-Jeffries, & David, 1990).

Thus, our findings raise disturbing questions about the relationship between ethnicity, schizophrenia, and criminal conviction. No doubt excess social deprivation and bias within the criminal justice system account for some of this. However, the study also raises the possible contribution of illness-related factors, particularly in young African-Caribbeans with schizophrenia.

CONCLUSION

We have confirmed and extended recent findings of an increased risk of criminal conviction in those with schizophrenia, particularly for assaultive offending in men. However, whilst we have added to the modern literature suggesting that serious mental illness is an independent risk factor for serious offending, it is important that this result is seen in context, both nationally and internationally.

First, as Coid has pointed out, whilst rates of "normal" homicide show dramatic inter country variations, those of "abnormal" homicide do not. This can lead to an erroneous impression of a high risk posed by the mentally ill in the a country such as UK in which the overall homicide rate is low (Coid, 1983). Second, the risk we and others have observed is small. Viewed in terms of attributable risk, the contribution made by those with schizophrenia to the level of recorded crime in the community is slender. Swanson et al. (1990) calculate that the relative risk of a limited range of self-reported violent behaviours in those with only schizophrenia or schizophreniform disorder is four, a substantial figure. However, the population attributable risk percentage (PAR%) can be obtained from their data, and is 3%. This implies that although being diagnosed with schizophrenia means that recall of violent behaviour is increased fourfold, such illnesses are associated with only 3% of all recorded violent behaviours. Link et al. (1992) came to a similar conclusion in their community sample. An alternative way of addressing the same question can be provided directly from our sample. Between 1964 and 1990, the last year of the study, the individuals with schizophrenia who form the basis of this book were in the community for a total of 7800 years following the onset of their illness, excluding time in hospital or prison. During those 7800 years there was a single homicide. This was the first psychiatric presentation of a middle-aged man, who was not previously known to any psychiatric service. We wonder just how often homicide by the severely mentally ill is preventable; this case certainly was not.

Third, we concluded that schizophrenia per se, the experience of mental illness, did contribute to the pattern of offending. We also found that substance abuse played a significant role. However, gender, ethnicity, age of onset, and previous offending all contributed more. No amount of psychiatric care or supervision can alter these associations.

CHAPTER EIGHT

Trends in the incidence of the functional psychoses

TRENDS IN THE INCIDENCE OF SCHIZOPHRENIA

Temporal trends in the incidence of a disease may provide valuable clues to its aetiology, especially with regard to changes in environmental risk factors. In recent years, a number of studies from developed countries have reported a possible decrease in the treated incidence of schizophrenia. Studies reporting such a decrease used national or regional admission data from Scotland (Dickson & Kendell, 1986; Eagles & Whalley, 1985; Geddes, Black, Whalley, & Eagles, 1993; Kendell, Malcolm, & Adams, 1993), England (Der, Gupta, & Murray, 1990), Australia (Parker, O'Donnell, & Walters, 1985), New Zealand (Joyce, 1987), and Denmark (Munk-Jørgensen, 1986; Munk-Jørgensen & Mortensen, 1993). Similar declines were reported in two UK studies which used first-contact data in smaller areas with a case register (De Alarçon, Seagroatt, & Goldacre, 1990; Eagles, Hunter, & McCance, 1988). On the other hand, studies using first admission data that reported no change or an increase in the treated incidence have come from France (Van Os et al., 1993) and Croatia (Folnegovic, Folnegovic-Šmalc, & Kulcar, 1990), whereas three studies which used first-contact data from case registers reported no change; one from Germany (Hafner & Gattaz, 1991) and three from the UK (Bamrah et al., 1991; Harrison, Cooper, & Gancarczyk, 1991).

The search for temporal trends in multifactorial disorders such as schizophrenia is a hazardous affair because of their variable clinical expression, course, and outcome. The most important methodological issues with regard to temporal trends in the incidence of psychosis are summarised in Table 8.1. A number of the studies examining trends in the incidence of schizophrenia have attempted to avoid these methodological pitfalls. Notably, some studies adjusted rates for the age and sex composition of the source population (e.g. Der et al., 1990, De Alarçon et al., 1990). Others used first-contact rates as opposed to studies on first-admission rates to avoid any artifact induced by a reduction in available hospital beds; similarly, quality of registration may affect nationwide registration systems, but is unlikely to affect smaller areas with a well-staffed case register.

Nevertheless, several problems remain (Kendell et al., 1993). First, there is the possibility that temporal changes in incidence rates might simply reflect changes in diagnostic criteria for the disease because of the highly variable clinical picture and the ephemeral nature of diagnostic concepts. Waddington and Youssef (1994) tried to circumvent this problem by calculating incidence of schizophrenia in birth cohorts rather than age cohorts. They assessed all cases of schizophrenia, using operationalised criteria, in a well-circumscribed geographical area, and calculated incidence of schizophrenia in successive birth cohorts of individuals born between 1920 and 1969. The problem, however, was their use of the morbid risk method to adjust for differences in disease expectancy in different birth cohorts: as the very assumption of the morbid risk method is that age-specific incidence rates are constant over time, this approach cannot, by definition, be used to resolve the issue of changing incidence over time.

Second, temporal changes in the incidence of a disorder may not be related only to changes in the age and sex composition of the source population, but also to changes in the ethnic composition (Harrison et al., 1991). Third, there may be concurrent changes in age of onset, which may present as changes in the incidence: for example, progressively earlier age of onset will lead to a spurious, apparent increase in the incidence of a disorder.

THE CURRENT STUDY

The Camberwell Register sample allowed us to examine trends in the incidence of the functional psychoses over an extended period, avoiding some of the methodological pitfalls outlined above. In particular, we ensured diagnostic uniformity by rediagnosing all cases according to contemporary criteria for psychosis (see Chapter 2), and we ascertained all contacts (not just admissions) with the psychiatric services of the defined

TABLE 8.1
Possible Factors Leading Changes In The Incidence Of Schizophrenia Based On
First-Admission Rates Or First-Contact Rates

Factor	Effect on first-contact or first-admission incidence	Mechanism
Reduction in number of psychiatric beds; development of community services and primary care services (1, 2, 3, 4)	Decline	Milder cases treated in the community; or increase in proportion of untreated cases due to pressure on services; or increased propoprtion treated in primary care; or delay in first treatment resulting in effective *later* age of first treatment over a period resulting in spurious decline in incidence (see also below at "change in age of onset").
Change in diagnostic habits (5, 6, 7, 8, 9)	Decline	Prevailing diagnostic criteria get more "narrow"; or clinicians get increasingly reluctant to diagnose schizophrenia at first onset; or chose a more "treatable" diagnostic label such as manic-depressive psychosis.
Change in diagnostic habits (10)	Increase	Prevailing diagnostic criteria get "wider".
Changes in ethnic composition of source population (11)	Increase	High rates of schizophrenia in some ethnic groups.
Changes in age of onset with time (7, 12)	Decline/increase	Earlier age of onset over a period will present as increase in incidence; the reverse will be the case with later age of onset (or age at first treatment, see above [5]).
Changes in age structure of source population (7)	Decline	A decline in the proportion of individuals in the age range most at risk will lead to spurious decline of incidence *if* study is not age standardised.
Changes in the quality of registration	Decline	Reductions in administrative manpower may lead to less accurate registration of treated incidence.
Real change in incidence (5, 12)	Decline	Change in incidence of risk factors, operating at the time of birth and/or at the time of disease onset.
Small area studies: differential mobility of (genetically) predisposed (13)	Decline/increase	Individuals at risk of schizophrenia drifting into deprived, inner-city areas, and movement of healthy individuals out of area will result in higher incidence.

1. Eagles (1993); Munk-Jørgensen & Mortensen (1993); 3. Prince & Phelan (1990); 4. Goldacre et al. (1994); 5. Der et al. (1990); 6. Crow (1990); 7. Kendell et al. (1993); 8. Parker et al. (1985); 9. Munk-Jørgensen (1987); 10. Van Os et al. (1993); 11. Harrison et al. (1991); 12. Eagles et al. (1988); 13. De Alarçon et al. (1990).

catchment area population of Camberwell over the period 1965 to 1984 (as outlined in Chapter 2). These analyses represent an updated and expanded version of those presented in Castle, Wessely, Der, and Murray (1991).

For the current analyses, we confined ourselves to RDC and DSM-III-R criteria for psychotic disorders. An adjustment was made for the missing notes, by ascertaining the percentage of rated patients (by sex and/or ethnicity where necessary) in each cohort, with a register diagnosis of schizophrenia and related conditions, who fulfilled RDC and DSM-III-R criteria for schizophrenia; this proportion was then added to the total in each category (these corrections resulted in only minor changes). Incidence rates for RDC schizophrenia were calculated, based on the census figures for the population of Camberwell, directly standardised to the 1964 age and sex structure.

Changes in rates over time were analysed with a test for trend for incidence rate ratios, using the Poisson regression procedure in the STATA statistical programme (STATA, 1995). In Poisson regression, the logarithm of the rate is the "response" variable, and the effects of a range of "explanatory" variables on the rate can be examined. The exponentiated regression coefficient for a given explanatory variable equals the rate ratio, i.e. the rate in the "exposed" group divided by the baseline rate. A series of models were fitted with time (measured in four five-year periods between 1965 and 1984, to allow for a time trend of incidence rates), gender, and age (eight groups) as the "explanatory" variables. Time was fitted by including a simple linear term ("period"). Age-by-period and gender-by-period interaction terms were fitted and evaluated with the Likelihood Ratio Statistic (LRS), to examine whether there was significant heterogeneity in the effect of time period at the different levels of gender or age. Associations between binary variables were expressed as the risk ratio (Rothman, 1986).

Sample period 1965–1984

Patients were allocated to four time cohorts, according to their date of first contact, namely 1965–69 (first cohort), 1970–74 (second cohort), 1975–79 (third cohort), and 1980–84 (fourth cohort). The number of patients in each cohort for whom notes were missing was 19 (14%), 22 (17%), 11 (8%), and 3 (2%). The greater proportion of missing notes in the first and second cohorts is because a number of these notes were destroyed because of lack of storage space at one of the local hospitals. There is no reason to suspect that this introduced any systematic bias; specifically, there were no significant differences in the proportion of males, or those born outside the UK, between persons with missing and available notes. An adjustment for missing notes was made as described above.

Trends in incidence

Table 8.2 shows the number of individuals over the period 1965–84 who fulfilled ICD criteria for study inclusion (ICD = 295.0–295.9, 297.2, 298.1–298.9). Visual inspection of the rates of RDC, DSM-III–R and ICD schizophrenia indicated an increase in the first-contact incidence over the period 1965–84, although this failed to achieve statistical significance (Figs 8.1–8.3). The first-admission incidence of RDC schizophrenia over the period 1965–92 similarly tended to increase (Fig. 8.4).

Effect of age and gender

There was no evidence that the effect of time period was modified by gender. However, for both first-contact rates over the period 1965–84, and for first-admission rates over the period 1965–92, an interaction with age of onset was apparent (Figs 8.1–8.4), such that there was a significant increase in incidence rates in the youngest age groups, but not in the older age groups (Table 8.3).

Ethnic group

To investigate any effect of ethnicity on our results, we established, among the total number of individuals fulfilling RDC criteria for schizophrenia, the proportion of both Caribbean-born and UK-born African-Caribbeans (Table 8.4). As detailed in Chapter 2, census data for Camberwell show that the proportion of the population born in the West Indies increased from 2.5% in 1961, to 4.9% in 1971, and 6.6% in 1981. The 1981 census also classifies residents by the birthplace of the head of the household. This can be used as a rough estimate of the proportion of the total

TABLE 8.2

Numbers Of Individuals Fulfilling Various Criteria For Schizophrenia, By Cohort

Cohort	Psychosis*	RDC†	DSM-III–R†	ICD†‡
1965–69	132	79 (60%)	50 (38%)	102 (77%)
1970–74	133	91 (68%)	55 (41%)	116 (87%)
1975–79	143	97 (68%)	60 (42%)	128 (89%)
1980–84	133	88 (66%)	53 (40%)	118 (89%)

   * Taken akin to a register diagnosis of "schizophrenic psychosis" (ICD codes 295.0–295.9), including schizoaffective type (ICD 295.7), "paraphrenia" (ICD 297.2) or "other non-organic psychosis" (ICD 298.1–298.9).
   † Numbers are adjusted for missing notes (see text).
   ‡ Taken akin to an ICD register diagnosis of 295.0–2.95.9 or 297.2.
   (Reprinted, with permission, from Castle et al., 1991.)

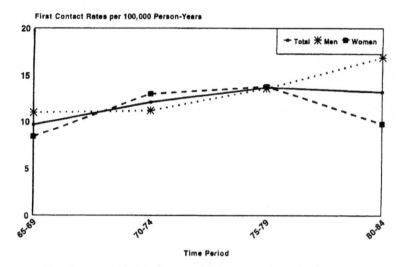

First Contact Rates per 100,000 Person-Years

Test for trend: Summary Incidence Rate Ratio over Four Periods: 1.1 (0.9-1.2); P=0.3
Gender-period interaction: Chi-square=0.9, P=0.3
Age-period interaction: Chi-square=3.4, P=0.06

FIG. 8.1. Five-year first-contact rates for RDC schizophrenia per 100,000 person-years, 1965–1984.

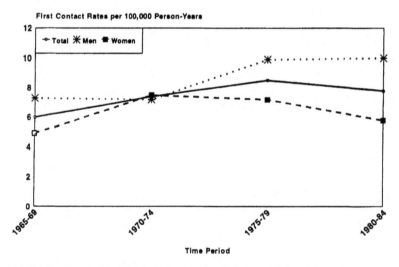

First Contact Rates per 100,000 Person-Years

Test for trend: Summary Incidence Rate Ratio over Four Periods: 1.0 (0.9-1.2); P=0.7
Gender-period interaction: Chi-square=0.4, P=0.5
Age-period interaction: Chi-square=3.4, P=0.07

FIG. 8.2. Five-year first-contact rates for DSM-III–R schizophrenia per 100,000 person-years, 1965–1984.

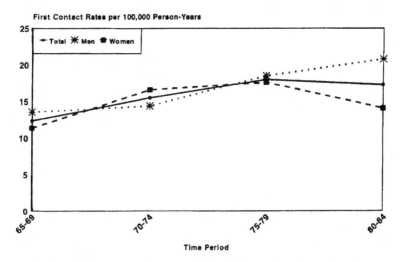

Test for trend: Summary Incidence Rate Ratio over Four Periods: 1.1 (0.97-1.0); P=0.2
Gender-period interaction: Chi-square=1.2, P=0.3
Age-period interaction: Chi-square=6.7, P=0.01

FIG. 8.3.   Five-year first-contact rates for ICD non-affective psychosis per 100,000 person-years, 1965–1984.

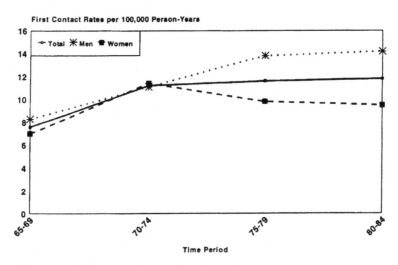

Test for trend: Summary Incidence Rate Ratio over Four Periods: 1.2 (1.1-1.3); P<0.01
Gender-period interaction: Chi-square=1.4, P=0.2
Age-period interaction: Chi-square=5.1, P=0.02

FIG. 8.4.   Five-year first-contact rates for RDC schizophrenia per 100,000 person-years, 1965–1984.

TABLE 8.3
Trends In The Incidence Of First-Contact Schizophrenia In The Period 1965–1984,
And First-Admission Schizophrenia In The Period 1965–1992, Camberwell, South
London

	1965–84* Summary IRR‡ (95% CI)	1965–92† Summary IRR‡ (95% CI)
Age group <25 years	1.2 (1.02–1.4)¶	1.5 (1.3–1.7)‖
Age group 25–44 years	1.0 (0.9–1.2)	1.1 (0.9–1.3)
Age group 45–64 years	1.0 (0.8–1.3)	0.9 (0.7–1.1)
Age group >64 years	0.9 (0.7–1.2)	1.0 (0.8–1.3)

* Divided into four five-year periods.
† Divided into four seven-year periods.
‡ The incidence rate ratio for shifting one period. For example, the summary IRR of 1.5 indicates that with each consecutive time period, the incidence increases with a factor 1.5. Thus, over four time periods, the incidence increases with a factor $1.5^3 = 3.4$.
¶ $P = .03$
‖ $P < .001$

population who were ethnic African-Caribbeans (i.e. those born in the West Indies, and those born in the UK combined); the figure for 1981 was 11.5% African-Caribbean. To avoid error through possible underestimation of the size of the African-Caribbean population, all denominator data for the group born in the West Indies and the African-Caribbean group were corrected for a 10% (King et al., 1994; Siegel, 1974) under-enumeration in all the analyses comparing ethnic groups (Table 8.5).

It is clear (Table 8.4) that the proportion of Caribbean-born individuals among participants with a diagnosis of RDC schizophrenia is five to six times higher than the proportion in the general population of Camberwell. In the later years of the study, a similar excess is seen for the African-Caribbean group as a whole (i.e. both Caribbean-born and UK-born).

Using the census data, corrected as described above, we calculated rates for RDC schizophrenia by country of birth (Table 8.5). The rate of

TABLE 8.4
Proportion Of All Individuals Fulfilling RDC Criteria For Schizophrenia,
By Country Of Birth And Ethnicity

Cohort	Individuals born in the West Indies	First and second generation African-Caribbeans
1965–69	13%	25%
1970–74	32%	38%
1975–79	30%	38%
1980–84	25%	40%

(Reprinted, with permission, from Castle et al., 1991.)

TABLE 8.5
Five-Year Rates (Rate Ratios) Of RDC Schizophrenia Per 100,000 Person-Years, By Country Of Birth*

Cohort		Individuals born in the West Indies	All individuals born in the UK	All African-Caribbeans	All other ethnic groups
1964–69	Number of cases‡	9.3	52.5	—	—
	Denominator*†	22961.0	776987.0	—	—
	Five-year rates	40.5	6.8	—	—
	Rate ratio (95% CI)	6.0 (3.0-12.0)		—	—
1970–74	Number of cases‡	23.8	52.4	—	—
	Denominator*†	40284.0	642025.0	—	—
	Five-year rates	59.1	8.2	—	—
	Rate ratio (95% CI)	7.2 (4.5-11.8)		—	—
1975–79	Number of cases‡	20.6	61.8	—	—
	Denominator*†	36307.0	578639.0	—	—
	Five-year rates	56.7	10.7	—	—
	Rate ratio (95% CI)	5.3 (3.2-8.7)		—	—
1980–84	Number of cases‡	17.4	59.3	31.3	56.2
	Denominator*†	45144.0	491251.0	78660.0	544809.0
	Five-year rates	38.5	12.1	39.8	10.3
	Rate ratio (95% CI)	3.2 (1.9-5.4)		3.9 (2.5-6.0)	

* Excludes all those born in neither the UK nor in the West-Indies.
† The denominator for population born in the West Indies, and "all African-Caribbeans" was corrected for an estimated 10% underenumeration.
‡ Decimal points resulting from minor corrections for missing case notes.
(Based on Castle et al., 1991.)

schizophrenia for "all individuals born in the West Indies" was significantly greater than that for "all individuals born in the UK", across all four time bands. Of course, in the later years of the study an increasing proportion of the general population in Camberwell were ethnic African-Caribbeans born in the UK; this probably accounts for the decline in the rate ratio for "country of birth" from the second to the fourth cohort. The limitations of the census data allow us to estimate rates by ethnicity as such only for the final five years of the study (again, "country of birth of head of household" data were used). Table 8.5 shows that for 1980–84, the rate of RDC schizophrenia for all ethnic African-Caribbeans was nearly four times that for all other ethnic groups combined (the great majority of whom would be white).

As the exact age structure of the African-Caribbean population in Camberwell over the period under investigation is not known, but is likely to have contained relatively few individuals in the older age groups compared to the white population, we attempted to correct for this effect. In our sample, age of onset distribution curves for African-Caribbeans and "all other ethnicities" were similar in form, but the range in African-Caribbeans was 16–62 years, and 16–89 years in the "all other ethnicities" sample. We therefore calculated, for the 1980–84 cohort, rates for "all other ethnicities" with onset before 65, assuming that all individuals in the general population in Camberwell aged 65 and over were white, to obtain a more conservative estimate of rate ratios between African-Caribbeans and "all other ethnicities" in the under-65s. With this correction, however, individuals of African-Caribbean origin showed rates of schizophrenia that were even higher as compared to their white counterparts (RR = 4.4; 95% CI = 2.7–7.0), the reason being that rates of schizophrenia in "all other ethnicities" were especially high after age 65, due to the large number of

TABLE 8.6
Age Distribution Of African-Caribbean Patients And Other Patients With An RDC Diagnosis Of Schizophrenia

Age group	Other groups*	African-Caribbean group*
<25 year	51 (22%)	46 (53%)
25–34 year	53 (23%)	18 (21%)
35–44 year	28 (12%)	10 (11%)
45–54 year	22 (9%)	10 (11%)
55–64 year	25 (11%)	3 (4%)
65–74 year	27 (12%)	0
75+ year	27 (12%)	0

Chi-square = 44.5, df = 6, P < .001.
* Numbers are not corrected for missing case-records.

cases of first contact schizophrenia in elderly women. Exclusion of this group would therefore result in lower rates in the "all other ethnicities" group.

In order to examine whether the above reported finding of an increase in incidence over the period 1965–84, which was confined to the youngest age group, was related to the finding that African-Caribbeans were at increased risk of schizophrenia, we compared the age distributions of African-Caribbean and other patients with RDC schizophrenia. There were significant differences in the age distributions, such that over 50% of the African-Caribbean patients, versus only around 20% of patients in the other groups, were younger than 25 years (RR = 2.4; 95% CI = 1.8–3.3; Table 8.6). This difference was constant over the four time periods.

DISCUSSION

Over the 20-year period from 1965 we found that there was evidence for an increase in the incidence of schizophrenia in Camberwell. This increase, however, was confined to the younger age groups of men and women; rates did not change in the older age groups. The African-Caribbean group was at greater risk of developing schizophrenia (RR = 3.9; 95% CI = 2.5–6.0), even after approximate adjustment for age and a 10% underestimation of the size of the African-Caribbean population in Camberwell.

Methodological issues

The use of first-contact rather than first-admission patients avoids the possibility of bias due to changes in admission policies over the years. Furthermore, the results were similar regardless of whether first contacts or first admissions were examined. However, our data were derived from service-based frequency statistics, which cannot register changes in referral patterns from primary care. It is, for example, theoretically possible that general practitioners in Camberwell have changed their pattern of referral of psychotic patients to psychiatric services, treating more and more patients themselves. The available evidence in the UK, however, suggests that almost all patients with severe mental illness are eventually referred to psychiatric services (Cooper et al., 1987). For example, Bamrah and colleagues (1991) found that only 7 out of 557 identified schizophrenic patients were solely in contact with their general practitioner. Further-more, even if such a change was operating, it would probably result, if anything, in a lower proportion of such patients being referred to hospital in more recent years (see Prince & Phelan, 1990), and thus cannot readily explain the increase in incidence we encountered. Since we assessed the widest feasible range of diagnoses on the register, it is unlikely that we omitted any significant number of schizophrenia patients among those who had psychiatric contact.

The study used diagnoses recorded at first-ever contact, and therefore excluded patients with, for example, affective disorder who later developed schizophrenia. However, we also screened 56 (75%) of the 75 "manic" patients on the register between 1971 and 1985, and rediagnosed them according to RDC criteria; only two patients fulfilled RDC criteria for schizophrenia. As an additional check for any schizophrenia patients we might have missed, we screened 80% of the patients on the register in the "paranoia" and "morbid jealousy" categories, and found no patients who fulfilled RDC criteria for schizophrenia. Furthermore, during the conduct of an accompanying case control study (see Chapter 7), the case records of 574 individuals, matched for age, sex and time period, and who were not in the "schizophrenia" categories of the register, were scrutinised. Only two of these were rediagnosed as "definite" schizophrenia by RDC criteria, and a further two were "possible" RDC schizophrenia according to the OPCRIT program.

Interpretation of findings

The trend in first-contact incidence over the period 1965–84 concurred with the trend in first-admission incidence over the period. A similar correspondence in results for first-admission rates and first-contact rates (though in that case a decline) was reported from Scotland (Eagles et al., 1988; Eagles & Whalley, 1985), although there was only limited overlap in the geographical areas studied. The similarity in change of first-contact and first-admission rates do suggest, however, that studies from New South Wales, New Zealand, England, Scotland, Croatia, France, and Denmark (Der et al., 1990; Eagles & Whalley, 1985; Folnegovic & Folnegovic-Šmalc, 1992; Joyce, 1987; Munk-Jørgensen & Mortensen, 1993; Parker et al., 1985; Van Os et al., 1993), which used national or regional data on first admissions may not be flawed because of changing service provisions over the periods of investigation.

In our study, there was an increase in incidence in the younger age groups, regardless of which data were used. Results were similar regardless of whether we used operationalised diagnoses or the clinical register diagnoses. It is unlikely, therefore, that diagnostic bias was operating to cause the temporal trend, as has been suggested for other studies by several investigators (Crow, 1990; Kendell et al., 1993; Van Os et al., 1993).

What could explain the disparity of results between our study suggesting a possible increase in the incidence of schizophrenia, and other studies discussed above which reported a decline? In examining possible factors we will focus on the studies that are most comparable with our own, that is, studies that were based on case register data from a small geographic area, and were conducted in the UK. Our results concur with one other UK register-based study (Harrison et al., 1991), but differ from two others, which showed a decline in rates for schizophrenia (De Alarçon et al., 1990; Eagles et al., 1988). It should be pointed out, however, that none of these other studies simultaneously allowed for age, gender, and ethnic group in the calculation of rates, all of which may be relevant to changes in the incidence of schizophrenia.

Changes in the age and sex structure of the general population. Changes in the age and sex structure may affect temporal changes in incidence rates if results are not adjusted for age and sex. However, failure to adjust for age and gender cannot explain disparities between these studies, as both the present study, and the study by De Alarçon and colleagues (1990) and Eagles and colleagues (1988) adjusted for changes in demographic characteristics, yet obtained opposite results.

Changes in the socioeconomic structure of the population. Is it possible that an overall decline in incidence in the UK was masked in Camberwell by changes in the socioeconomic structure of the population? Camberwell is an inner city area with high levels of socioeconomic deprivation and unemployment, which has been rising over the period under investigation. There has also been a general decline in the total population in Camberwell over the same period. It is well known that the treated incidence of psychiatric disorders (including psychotic disorders) is associated, at least at the ecological level, with the level of socioeconomic deprivation in inner city areas (reviewed by Cooper et al., 1987; Freeman, 1994). Although census figures show that there was only a slight increase in the proportion of Camberwell residents in social classes IV and V between 1971 and 1981 (27.3% in 1971; 28.6% in 1981), there was a modest decrease and a lower baseline rate of individuals in classes IV and V in England as a whole (26.2.% in 1971; 23% in 1981). Thus, Camberwell is a deprived area relative to many parts of the country and, even if social class is an imperfect marker for socioeconomic deprivation, there has been a relative increase in deprivation over the period under investigation. Given the association between deprivation and treated incidence of schizophrenia, it is possible that the relative increase in deprivation over the period under investigation contributed to our finding of a rising incidence in the younger age groups (most at risk of developing schizophrenia). Those geographical areas which have reported a decline in the incidence of schizophrenia, such as Aberdeenshire and Oxfordshire, have become relatively more prosperous than Camberwell (De Alarçon et al., 1990; Eagles et al., 1988). However, given the modest association between level of deprivation and schizophrenia incidence in previous studies (Cooper et al., 1987; Torrey & Bowler, 1991), it is unlikely that the relatively minor changes in socioeconomic structure would explain the marked rise in incidence in the youngest age groups.

Changes in the ethnic composition. Harrison and colleagues (1991) reported that incidence rates for schizophrenia had been stable in Nottingham between 1975 and 1987. Although the rates were not adjusted for age, gender, or ethnic group, it was suggested that the discrepancy between constant incidence in Nottingham versus the decline in incidence in Aberdeen and Oxford (De Alarçon et al., 1990; Eagles et al., 1988) could be related to the greater proportion of ethnic minorities among the population of Nottingham, who in a previous study had been shown to be at high risk of developing psychosis (Harrison et al., 1988). To turn to our study, three lines of evidence suggest that the rise in incidence in the youngest age groups may be associated with the influx into Camberwell of (young) African-Caribbean individuals over the period under investigation: (1) African-Caribbean patients were relatively overrepresented in the youngest age groups; (2) African-Caribbean individuals were at substantially higher risk to develop schizophrenia; and (3) the proportion of African-Caribbeans among the population in Camberwell gradually increased over the period under investigation. It is therefore very possible that the rise in incidence in the younger age groups was largely determined by high rates in African-Caribbean individuals.

One might suspect that it is even possible that the constant incidence found in the older age groups in fact represented a decline in incidence which was obscured by the lesser effect of high rates in certain ethnic groups in the older age categories (as there were fewer Afro-Caribbean individuals in the older age groups, the effect of ethnicity on incidence rates over time would have been less pronounced). If the incidence in the white group had indeed declined, however, one would expect to find an indication of decreasing incidence in the oldest age groups, where the proportion of African-Caribbean individuals in the general population would have been very small. In Table 8.3, however, there is no such indication: in the highest age group of 64 years and older, in which no African-Caribbean patients (or patients from other ethnic groups who are at high risk of developing psychosis; King et al., 1994; Rwegerella, 1977) were present, the incidence appeared to remain constant over the period under investigation. These results are in concordance with the investigation by Der and colleagues, who reported that the substantial decrease in rates in England between 1952 and 1986 was limited to the younger age groups

(Der et al., 1990), whose disease may be aetiologically different from those with onset at a higher age (Castle & Howard, 1992; Van Os et al., 1995; and Chapter 6). Because of the inadequacies of the census information, it is difficult to examine further the effect of ethnic group in different age groups.

In conclusion, the rate of schizophrenia in Camberwell has increased in the youngest age groups over the period 1965–1986 and 1965–1992, and remained constant in the older age groups. We suggest that the main reason for the discrepancy with other studies showing a decrease in the incidence in younger age groups lies in the change in the ethnic composition of the source population in Camberwell over the two decades from the mid-1960s. Another likely contributing factor, though possibly of less impact, is the increase in social deprivation over the period under investigation.

TRENDS IN THE INCIDENCE OF MANIA

There have been conflicting reports about changes in the incidence of mania over the last few decades. Eagles and colleagues (1988) found that age-standardised first-contact rates of mania had not changed over the period 1969–1984 in a defined area in northeast Scotland (Eagles et al., 1988). A number of studies, however, have suggested increasing incidence rates for the illness. Parker and colleagues (1985), for example, found a 35% increase in first admission rates for mania between 1967 and 1977 in New South Wales, which they suggested was due to clinicians using this label more after the introduction of lithium for bipolar disorder. Similarly, Kendell and coworkers (1993) noted an increase in first admission rates for mania in females between 1971 and 1989 in Edinburgh. However, in England and Wales, Der and colleagues (1990) reported a decline in first admission rates for manic depressive psychosis between 1952 and 1986, without a compensatory increase in any other diagnostic category. A similar decline in first admission rates has also been found for manic depressive psychosis in France, especially in females, in the absence of a concurrent increase in other psychiatric diagnoses (Van Os et al., 1993). The latter two studies, however, did not distinguish between depression and mania, and none of the above studies could exclude the possibility of bias due to changing diagnostic habits, fluctuating proportions of "false" first admissions (i.e. patients labelled "first admission" who in effect had had previous psychiatric treatment elsewhere), or alterations in admission policies over the years (Kendell et al., 1993).

In the previous section, we reported that the incidence of operationally defined schizophrenia in the area of Camberwell, South London, tended to rise over the period 1965–84, especially in the younger age groups. We suggested that one reason for the disparity between this finding and a number of reports of a decline in first admission rates in the UK for schizophrenia over the same period (Der et al., 1990; Eagles & Whalley, 1985; Kendell et al., 1993), lay in the changes in the ethnic composition of Camberwell over the decades from the mid-1960s, specifically the increase in the proportion of African-Caribbeans, who presented at younger ages than their white counterparts. Evidence has accumulated that African-Caribbean individuals living in the UK have a higher risk of developing schizophrenia than do their white counterparts (Dean, Walsh, Downing, & Shelley, 1981; Harrison et al., 1988; McGovern & Cope, 1987; Rwegellera, 1977). Is this increased risk confined to schizophrenia? Leff, Fisher and Bertelsen (1976), examining the annual incidence of mania in Camberwell, found that first generation African-Caribbeans (i.e. Caribbean-born) had higher rates than did indigenous whites. Within the affective disorder spectrum, the increase in relative risk for African-Caribbeans in the UK may be confined to mania. For example, Bebbington, Hurry, and Tennant (1981) noted that mean age-corrected admission rates for mania were more than three times higher in first generation African-Caribbeans than in UK-born patients, but if all affective disorders were combined no clear ethnic difference was discernible. Der and Bebbington (1987) reported similar results.

However, there are a number of difficulties with these studies. The study by Leff and colleagues (1976) was the only one to use operational criteria for mania, but the sample included only hospital admissions. All studies excluded manic cases with schizophrenic "first rank" symptoms, and none included African-Caribbean individuals born in the UK (second generation), who instead were incorporated in the group of individuals "born in the UK" together with whites and other ethnic groups; in some of the studies, the number of African-Caribbeans was very small (e.g. only six in the study by Leff et al., 1976). Furthermore, an initial presentation bias may be operating. Previous studies did not include those individuals with a first presentation of depression who might subsequently have developed manic episodes, and there may exist ethnic differences in the proportion of manic patients who will present with previous depressive episodes (Makanjuola, 1985).

If indeed there is an increased risk for both mania and schizophrenia in African-Caribbean individuals in the UK, this would have important implications both for psychiatric service provision and for theories of aetiology. For example, a variety of social and biological factors has been suggested as explanations for the increased risk of schizophrenia in African-Caribbeans (Harrison, 1990; and Chapter 9). If the increased risk was not confined to schizophrenia, but was also evident in mania, this could suggest that the excess in incidence is determined by a risk factor common to both illnesses.

The aim of this study, then, was to explore time trends in the incidence rate for operationally defined mania in a delimited area, in relation to ethnic group. In view of the evidence indicating gender differences in time trends in the incidence of mania, rates for men and women were also compared. The data represent an extension of those presented in Van Os et al. (1996d).

THE CURRENT STUDY

Table 8.7 shows the number of individuals who fulfilled RDC criteria for mania with schizomania across the four cohorts ($n = 106$), the great majority of whom (89.4%), had been inpatients at first contact. Incidence rates were calculated for mania and mania with schizomania. Incidence rates tended to go up for both mania with schizomania and mania, but this trend was not significant (Fig. 8.5 and Fig. 8.6).

Gender and age at first contact interactions

There were no interactions with gender in the analyses with period as the exposure variable. Contrary to the analyses on schizophrenia incidence in the previous section, there was no interaction between age at first contact and time period (LRS = 0.01, $P = .9$).

TABLE 8.7

Numbers Of Individuals Fulfilling RDC Criteria For Mania With Schizomania, By Cohort, And Annual Incidence Rates For Mania And Mania With Schizomania, Standardised To The 1964 Age And Sex Structure

Cohort	Number of psychotic individuals examined	Number with RDC mania with schizomania	Rate per 100,000 person-years	
			Mania with schizomania**	Mania**
1965–69	156	23 (15%)	2.8	1.7
1970–74	152	25 (16%)	3.4	2.0
1975–79	163	30 (18%)	4.3	3.8
1980–84	154	28 (18%)	4.1	3.4
Test for trend			$P = .09$	$P = .1$

* Numbers are adjusted for missing notes, according to the percentage of individuals (in parenthesis) with a register diagnosis of 'schizophrenia', 'paraphrenia', 'mania' or 'other non-organic psychosis', who fulfilled RDC criteria for mania or schizomania.

** For definitions of mania and mania with schizomania, see text.

(Reprinted, with permission, from Van Os et al., 1996d.)

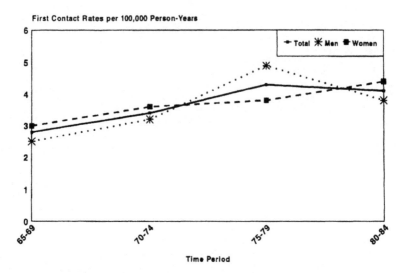

First Contact Rates per 100,000 Person-Years

Test for trend: Summary Incidence Rate Ratio over Four Periods: 1.1 (0.9-1.3); P=0.3
Gender-period interaction: Chi-square=0.4, P=0.5
Age-period interaction: Chi-square=0.01, P=0.9

FIG. 8.5. Five-year first-contact rates for RDC mania and schizomania per 100,000 person-years, 1965–1984.

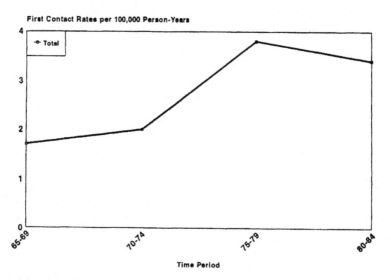

First Contact Rates per 100,000 Person-Years

Test for trend: P=0.3

FIG. 8.6. Five-year first-contact rates for RDC mania per 100,000 person years, 1965–1984.

100

Incidence of mania by ethnicity

In order to investigate any effect of ethnicity on our results, we established, among the total number of individuals fulfilling RDC criteria for mania with schizomania, the proportion of both Caribbean-born ($n = 22$) and UK-born African-Caribbeans ($n = 28$; Table 8.8). To avoid error through possible underestimation of the size of the African-Caribbean population, all denominator data for the group born in the West Indies and the African-Caribbean group were corrected for a 10% underenumeration in all the analyses comparing ethnic groups (Tables 8.9 and 8.10).

Using the census data, corrected as described, we calculated rates for RDC mania with schizomania by country of birth (Table 8.9). The rate of mania for "all individuals born in the West Indies" was significantly greater than that for "all individuals born in the UK", across all four time bands. Of course, in the later years of the study an increasing proportion of the general population in Camberwell were ethnic African-Caribbeans born in the UK; this probably accounts for the decline in the rate ratio for "country of birth" from the second to the fourth cohort. The limitations of the census data allowed us to estimate rates by ethnicity as such for the final five years of the study only (again, "country of birth of head of household" data were used). Table 8.9 shows that for 1980–84, the rate of mania for all ethnic African-Caribbeans was four times that for all other ethnic groups combined (the great majority of whom would be white).

Among all patients with mania, individuals in the African-Caribbean group were significantly more likely to fulfil criteria for "schizomania" than those in the white group ($RR = 2.2$; 95% $CI = 1.1$–4.3). Comparison of rates for mania (i.e. with exclusion of schizomania) in the 1980–84 cohort, by ethnicity, revealed a decrease in the rate ratio from 4.1 for mania with schizomania to 3.0 (95% $CI = 1.3$–7.4).

The exact age structure of the African-Caribbean population in Camberwell over the period under investigation is not known, but is

TABLE 8.8

Proportion Of All Individuals Fulfilling RDC Criteria For Mania With Schizomania, By Country Of Birth And Ethnicity

Cohort	Individuals born in the West Indies (n = 22)	First- and second- generation African-Caribbeans (n = 28)
1965–69	20%	21%
1970–74	23%	24%
1975–79	14%	21%
1980–84	25%	37%

(Reprinted, with permission, from Van Os et al., 1996d.)

TABLE 8.9
Five-Year Rates (Rate Ratios) Of RDC Mania With Schizomania Per 100,000 Person Years, By Country Of Birth*

Cohort		Individuals born in the West Indies	All individuals born in the UK	All African-Caribbeans	All other ethnic groups
1965–69	Number of cases‡	4.5	14.1	—	—
	Denominator†	22961.0	776987.0	—	—
	Five-year rates	19.6	1.8	—	—
	Rate ratio (95% CI)	10.8 (3.7,31.2)		—	—
1970–74	Number of cases‡	5.8	11.5	—	—
	Denominator†	40284.0	642025.0	—	—
	Five-year rates	14.4	1.8	—	—
	Rate ratio (95% CI)	8.0 (3.0,21.8)		—	—
1975–79	Number of cases‡	4.3	23.3	—	—
	Denominator†	36307.0	578639.0	—	—
	Five-year rates	11.8	4.0	—	—
	Rate ratio (95% CI)	2.9 (1.1,8.2)		—	—
1980–84	Number of cases‡	7.0	19.1	10.4	17.7
	Denominator†	45144.0	491251.0	78660.0	544809.0
	Five-year rates	15.5	3.9	13.2	3.3
	Rate ratio (95% CI)	4.0 (1.7,9.5)		4.1 (1.9,8.8)	

* Excludes all those born in neither the UK nor in the West Indies.

† The denominator for the population born in the West Indies and the African-Caribbean population was corrected for an estimated 10% underenumeration.

‡ Decimal points resulting from minor corrections for missing case notes.

CI confidence interval.

(Reprinted, with permission, from Van Os et al., 1996d.)

TABLE 8.10
Five-Year Rates (Rate Ratios) Of First Contact RDC Mania With Schizomania, And
First Admission Mania After Initial Depressive Episodes Per 100,000 Person Years, By
Country Of Birth*

Cohort		Individuals born in the West Indies	All individuals born in the UK
1965–69	Number of cases‡	10.5	35.1
	Denominator†	22961.0	776987.0
	Five-year rates	45.7	4.5
	Rate ratio (95% CI)	10.1 (5.1,20.2)	
1970–74	Number of cases‡	10.8	72.5
	Denominator†	40284.0	642025.0
	Five-year rates	26.8	11.3
	Rate ratio (95% CI)	2.4 (1.3,4.5)	
1975–79	Number of cases‡	9.3	60.3
	Denominator†	36307.0	578639.0
	Five-year rates	25.6	10.4
	Rate ratio (95% CI)	2.5 (1.2,4.9)	
1980–84	Number of cases‡	11.0	38.1
	Denominator†	45144.0	491251.0
	Five-year rates	24.4	7.8
	Rate ratio (95% CI)	3.1 (1.6,6.1)	

* Excludes all those born in neither the UK nor in the West Indies.
† The denominator for population born in the West Indies was corrected for an estimated 10% underenumeration.
‡ Decimal points resulting from minor corrections for missing case notes.
CI Confidence interval.
(Reprinted, with permission, from Van Os et al., 1996d.)

likely to have contained relatively few individuals in the older age groups compared to the white population. We attempted to correct for this effect. In our sample, age-at-onset distribution curves for African-Caribbeans and "all other ethnicities" were similar in form, but the range in African-Caribbeans was 16–64 years, and 16–88 years in the "all other ethnicities" sample. We therefore calculated, for the 1980–84 cohort, rates for "all other ethnicities" with onset before 65, assuming that all individuals in the general population in Camberwell aged 65 and over were white, to obtain a more conservative estimate of rate ratios between African-Caribbeans and "all other ethnicities" in the under 65s. With this correction, individuals of African-Caribbean origin showed rates of mania between 3.1 (mania with schizomania; 95% CI = 1.4–6.9), and 2.2 (mania; 95% CI = 0.9–5.6) times that of their white counterparts. Contrary to our findings in the patients with RDC schizophrenia described in the previous section, there was no evidence for a significant excess of African-Caribbean patients in the youngest age group (Table 8.11).

TABLE 8.11
Age Distribution Of African-Caribbean Patients And Other
Patients With An RDC Diagnosis Of Mania With
Schizomania.

Age group	Other groups*	African-Caribbean group*
<25 year	28 (41%)	7 (27%)
25–34 year	13 (19%)	11 (42%)
35–44 year	9 (13%)	3 (12%)
45–54 year	9 (13%)	4 (15%)
55–64 year	4 (6%)	1 (4%)
65–74 year	4 (6%)	0
75+ year	2 (3%)	0

Chi-square = 7.6, df = 6, P = .3.
* Numbers are not corrected for missing case-records.

Initial presentation bias?

As pointed out previously, one reason for the high rates of mania in African-Caribbeans may lie in differences in illness presentation: African-Caribbean bipolar patients possibly presenting more often with initial manic episodes, and bipolar white patients with initial depressive episodes.

To examine the possibility of differential change of diagnosis, we conducted a search for all patients on the Camberwell Case Register who had (1) an initial first-contact diagnosis of depression during the period 1965–1984, and (2) whose country of birth was either the UK (n = 2454; 91%) or the Caribbean (n = 239; 9%). This group of initial depressive contacts (IDC) was subsequently matched with computerised records of all discharges (including data on ICD discharge diagnosis and country of birth) to the Maudsley Hospital between 1970 and 1993, yielding a follow-up range for IDC cases from 5 to 28 years. This yielded matches with 2441 inpatient episodes, corresponding to 1481 patients (who could be matched more than once if they had multiple admissions). This group of 1481 had the same distribution of Caribbean-born and UK-born (Caribbean-born: n = 143, 10%; UK-born: n = 1338, 90%) as the whole IDC group, indicating an equal probability for both groups of being matched. Of the 1481 cases, a total of 335 patients (23%) had diagnoses in a non-depressive category, 158 of whom had a manic diagnosis, which is 11% of the 1481 matched patients, and 6% of the whole IDC group.

Contrary to expectation, Caribbean-born individuals were more likely to receive a follow-up diagnosis of mania (UK-born: n = 138/1338, Caribbean-born: n = 20/143, RR = 1.4; 95% CI = 0.9–2.1). Caribbean-born individuals were also more likely to receive a diagnosis of schizophrenia, schizoaffective disorder, paranoid psychosis or "other psychoses" (RR = 3.9; 95% CI = 2.4–6.3), especially schizophrenia (RR = 4.7; 95% CI = 2.7–8.2). However, Caribbean-born individuals were less likely to receive a follow-up diagnosis of neurosis or personality disorder (RR = 0.6; 95% CI = 0.4–0.9). If anything, these figures represent an underestimation of the true association between ethnic group and diagnostic change, as in the later years of the study an increasing proportion of the UK-born were ethnic African-Caribbeans born in the UK.

Adding the new figures of bipolars initially presenting as depressives to the cases of first-contact mania with schizomania, we recalculated the rates in both ethnic groups. In general, the rate ratio was only affected by a small amount, with the exception of the second cohort. In all four cohorts, however, rates remained significantly higher for the Caribbean-born group (Table 8.10). In view of the fact that Caribbean-born depressives were nearly four times more likely to receive a follow-up diagnosis of schizophrenia, it is clear that the presented rate ratios in the previous sections, if anything, represent an underestimation of the true effect size of ethnic group on the incidence of schizophrenia. Therefore, if the use of first contact or first admission diagnoses of schizophrenia is biased by differential diagnostic labelling of patients from different ethnic groups, the direction of the bias is to decrease the ethnic difference, rather than increase it.

DISCUSSION

Over the 20-year period from 1965 we found that there was some evidence for a rise in the incidence of mania in Camberwell. The African-Caribbean group was at greater risk of developing mania (rate ratio = 3.1; 95% CI = 1.4–6.9), after adjustment for age and a 10% underestimate of the size of the Afro-Caribbean population in Camberwell. Initial presentation bias is unlikely to have affected our results. Before considering these findings further, we need to discuss possible methodological flaws in our study, some of which have already been addressed.

The use of first-contact rather than first-admission patients avoids the possibility of bias due to changes in admission policies over the years. Although it is theoretically possible that general practitioners in Camberwell have changed their pattern of referral of manic patients to psychiatric services, the available evidence in the UK suggests that almost all patients with severe mental illness are referred to psychiatric services (Cooper et al., 1987). Furthermore, as argued in the previous section, even if such a change was operating, it would probably result, if anything, in a lower proportion of such patients being referred to hospital in more recent years (see Prince & Phelan, 1990). Again, we assessed the widest feasible range of diagnoses on the register, and it is unlikely that we omitted any significant number of manic patients.

We have shown that exclusion of bipolar patients with first episodes of depression is unlikely to have led to spurious results. Although diagnostic change from depression to mania was only evaluated for cases on the register who had subsequent admissions to hospital, 90% of our first contact sample with manic disorder were inpatients, so that few manic patients with initial depressive episodes would have been missed. Our follow-up period to asses diagnostic change was long enough, as most of the conversion from depression to bipolar disorder takes place in the first five years of illness (Akiskal et al., 1995). The overall rate of change from depression to bipolar disorder in our study is somewhere between 6% (of initial first-contact depressives, a substantial portion of whom would have moved out of the area before suffering an affective relapse) and 11% (of those initial depressives who remained in the area and had further contact with services). This estimate is similar to figures in the recent NIMH 11-year follow-up study of major depressive disorder, which found that 3.9% of participants developed (manic) bipolar I disorder, and 8.6% (hypomanic) bipolar II disorder over the ensuing years (Akiskal et al., 1995). Given that many hypomanic episodes occurring in bipolar II disorder are unlikely to be diagnosed as such (e.g. mild hypomania of a few days' duration), and the predominant clinical picture in bipolar II disorder is of protracted depressive episodes (Akiskal et al., 1995), the overall conversion rate in the NIMH study (3.9% + 8.6% = 12.5%) would be much lower if the method of case detection had been similar to the one used in this investigation (as many bipolar II cases would have been missed).

Interpretation of findings

Overall, the rate for mania over the period under study tended to increase, although this may have arisen by chance. Our results do not indicate that the rate for mania has decreased. Kendell and colleagues (1993) claimed an increase in the rate of mania for women as opposed to men, but did not provide evidence of significant differences in rates between men and women. These authors ascribed their result to changing diagnostic habits, and the authors of another study reporting an increase in the incidence of mania (Parker et al., 1985) suggested that changes in diagnostic habits and changing proportions of "false" first admissions had contributed significantly to their results. The design of our present study, however, precluded bias due to changes in diagnostic habits at first contact, by using standardised operational criteria based on comprehensive case records, and systematic bias in the missing notes is unlikely. It is possible, however, that changes in the composition of the population of Camberwell over the period of the study have contributed to our findings. As already discussed, three major factors should be considered in this regard.

Changes in the age and sex structure of the general population. The rates for mania shown in Figs 4.5 and 4.6 are standardised to the age and sex structure of Camberwell in 1964, thus obviating any effect of the changing age and sex structure of the population. We also "corrected" conservatively for the relative youth of the African-Caribbean population in Camberwell, and this did not alter our results significantly.

Changes in the socioeconomic structure of the population. It has been reported that mania is evenly distributed between the social classes in Camberwell (Leff et al., 1976; Der & Bebbington, 1987). Furthermore, as detailed in Chapter 2, the minor changes in the socioeconomic structure of Camberwell over the period under study could not account for the magnitude of the changes in the incidence of major psychiatric disorders in Camberwell. Thus, this is unlikely to be a major factor in our study.

Changes in the ethnic composition. Our finding of an increased risk for mania in African-Caribbean individuals is consonant with earlier reports of a relative risk of four-six times in Caribbean-born individuals compared to UK-born individuals (Bebbington et al., 1981; Der & Bebbington, 1987; Leff et al., 1976).

It is not possible to determine exactly, however, whether high rates in the African-Caribbean group were the main determinant of the apparent increase in the incidence of mania over the study period. Because of the inadequacies of the census data, it is difficult to give precise rates of mania by ethnic grouping, and by both ethnic grouping and gender. On the basis of our earlier estimate that African-Caribbeans comprised 11.5% of the population in 1981, we calculated a rate for mania with schizomania of 3.3 per 100,000 person-years for all non-African-Caribbeans between 1980 and 1984. Table 8.9 shows that the rate of mania with schizomania was 1.8 per 100,000 person-years for the general population for 1965–69. At this time there would have been very few UK-born African-Caribbeans in the population entering the age at risk for mania, as the major influx from the West Indies was in the 1950s and 1960s. The rate of 1.8 for "all individuals born in the UK" in the 1965–69 cohort was lower than the rate of 3.3 for "all non-African-Caribbeans" in the 1980–84 cohort (RR = 1.8; 95% CI = 0.9–3.7). Thus, this difference suggests that, independent of the growth of the African-Caribbean population in Camberwell, the rate of mania with schizomania was rising. This contrasts with the results on schizophrenia in the previous section, and would explain why, in the analyses with mania, no interaction was found between the effect of time period and age of onset, which in the previous section we interpreted as evidence of an ethnic group-dependent increase in incidence. It should be noted, however, that the 1965–69 rate for "all individuals born in the UK" is not strictly comparable to the 1980–84 rate for "all non-African-Caribbeans", as the latter includes a small number of immigrants from Africa who might also have a particular susceptibility to mania (Rwegellera, 1977).

In the entire sample, African-Caribbean individuals, and especially females, were more likely than their white counterparts to fulfil criteria for schizomania and, correspondingly, there was a decline in the rate ratio for "all African-Caribbeans" versus "all other ethnicities" if schizomania was excluded. Thus, African-Caribbeans with mania more frequently displayed "schizophrenic" symptomatology, and an excess of mixed affective and schizophrenic states, particularly in women, contributed to the increased risk of mania in African-Caribbeans.

CONCLUSIONS

The analyses in the first section of this chapter focused on the incidence of schizophrenia. While no definite conclusions about changes in the incidence could be drawn, there was support for the suggestion that changes in the incidence were related to changes in the ethnic composition of the source population. We have now demonstrated a similar relationship with regard to the incidence of mania, although there may have been a rise in the incidence of mania independent of changes in the ethnic composition of the source population. Ethnicity in relation to major mental illness is explored further in the following two chapters, first through the use of a case–control design (Chapter 9), and then by use of the 1991 census data to establish more accurate denominators data in respect to ethnicity (Chapter 10).

CHAPTER NINE

A case control study of ethnicity and schizophrenia

The data presented in Chapter 8 highlight the marked discrepancy in rates of functional psychosis in individuals of Caucasian and of African-Caribbean descent in Camberwell. To investigate this finding further, we performed a matched case–control study, using non-psychotic controls from the same Register as the cases. Before describing this study, an overview of the relevant literature is presented.

During the 1970s and 1980s several studies suggested that the rate of schizophrenia in the African-Caribbean population in the UK is higher than that those found in non-African-Caribbean samples (Bebbington et al., 1981; Cochrane & Bal, 1989; Harvey, Williams, McGuffin, & Toone, 1990; Rwegellera, 1977). This increase is found also in the children of African-Caribbean migrants, and some studies suggest that the second generation has an even higher rate of schizophrenia than their parents (Harrison et al., 1988; McGovern & Cope, 1987).

However, no single study is methodologically satisfactory. Several depend upon the routinely collected data of the Mental Health Enquiry (Cochrane & Bal, 1989; Glover, 1989a). Such data have a number of limitations. Definitions of schizophrenia are unstandardised, place of birth is not always recorded, and ethnicity rarely, thus excluding all those of African-Caribbean ethnicity born in the UK. Finally, data concern only hospital admissions.

McGovern and Cope (1987) recorded ethnicity as well as place of birth, but were still restricted to inpatients, and did not use operationally defined

109

criteria for schizophrenia. Only two studies used direct interviews and standardised criteria (Harrison et al., 1988; Harvey et al., 1990), of which only the study by Harrison and colleagues was population based. However, the power of that study was limited by the small sample size. Of the 28 cases of schizophrenia in African-Caribbeans, 18 were born in the UK and 10 in the Caribbean. Of the latter, only 2 had come to the UK after the age of 18. Nevertheless, despite the small sample size, the 95% confidence limit for the rate ratios for schizophrenia in African-Caribbeans compared to non-African-Caribbeans had a lower limit of six, a substantial excess (Harrison, 1990).

Problems also exist in calculating appropriate denominators, as outlined in Chapters 2 and 8. Before the 1991 Census, no accurate figures existed of the size of the African-Caribbean population in the UK. Reliable statistics are only available for place of birth, not ethnicity, and even then it has been suggested that many young blacks of both British and Caribbean birth did not register for either the 1971 or 1981 Census (Cruickshank & Beevers, 1989). One solution has been to use data concerning the head of household, and to assume that all those recorded as UK born but living in the household of someone recorded as being born in the Caribbean are second generation African-Caribbeans. However, this may considerably underestimate the size of the second generation population, since it assumes that all second generation children remain in the same household, and that all those resident in the household are of similar ethnic origin. The absence of reliable data about the size and age structure of the African-Caribbean population means that it remains possible that the apparent increase in schizophrenia is at least in part due to increasing numbers of young African-Caribbeans in the population and age at risk, rather than a true increase in age standardised rates.

The data presented in Chapter 8 go some way towards answering these criticisms, in that we used standardised diagnostic criteria, and ascertained all contacts rather than just admissions. The use of the 1991 Census data allowed a more accurate estimation of the denominator, but, for reasons outlined in Chapter 10, there are strong reasons to suspect under-estimation of ethnic minority groups even in the 1991 Census. Therefore, we decided to employ a different strategy, that of a case–control design (Schlesselman, 1982).

THE CURRENT STUDY

In this study individuals with schizophrenia (cases) are compared to those without schizophrenia but with other mental disorders (controls), with respect to a particular attribute (ethnicity). As such, this work represents an extension of that presented in Castle, Der, & Murray (1991).

The selection of cases is the same as for the previous chapters. As before, cases were all patients with first-contact schizophrenia and related conditions in Camberwell, SE London, between 1964 and 1984, as listed by the Camberwell Psychiatric Case Register. For these analyses, we used three different sets of diagnostic criteria (ICD-9, RDC, DSM-III-R), obtained via the OPCRIT programme. This was to address the suggestion made by some authors (e.g. Littlewood & Lipsedge, 1982), that some African-Caribbeans labelled as having schizophrenia in fact have a milder good-outcome form of psychotic illness. As this is a study of risk, and not rates, no corrections are made for missing data.

Controls were selected from the same register. A control was the next person on the register to a case, matched for sex and age (to within five years). Controls were therefore matched for time period.

Place of birth and ethnicity were obtained from case records. The general standard of case record keeping was high, and nearly all contained information on ethnicity in either the medical or nursing notes. In cases of doubt, further information was obtained either from the Maudsley Hospital computerised record system, which now records ethnicity, or general practitioner records. Those in whom the parents were of different ethnic origins were classified according to the description contained in the case records: only two were found, both classified as African-Caribbean.

No adequate data could be obtained on ethnicity for 19 controls, usually since they had made only brief contact with one particular local outpatient department which has since destroyed their records. These were replaced by new controls. Two checks were made on the reliability of the recording of ethnicity. As part of other studies, direct contemporary interviews that included recording ethnicity had been carried out for 34 patients, and other data sources that directly recorded ethnicity were available for a further 21 patients; no misclassifications were found. Four controls fulfilled criteria for schizophrenia and were thus replaced by new controls.

Place of birth was classified as follows: UK and Eire; West Indies; Asia; Africa; other. Ethnicity was classified as follows: Caucasian; African-Caribbean; Asian; other. In this chapter, we present analyses of African-Caribbeans alone: either born in the West Indies or born in the UK to parents born in the West Indies. Any patients born in Africa, and Asians born in the Caribbean, were not included as cases.

Classical analyses

The data were analysed by four time periods (1965–1969; 1970–1974; 1975–1979; 1980–1984). The traditional method of calculation is illustrated in Table 9.1. As the study is matched, only those pairs discordant for

TABLE 9.1
ICD Schizophrenia

Row	Matched pair	Period of presentation			
		1965–1969	1970–1974	1975–1979	1980–1984
1	Case Caucasian Control Caucasian	69	63	72	61
2	Case Caucasian Control African-Caribbean	6	6	2	4
3	Case African-Caribbean Control Caucasian	16	24	33	35
4	Case African-Caribbean Control African-Caribbean	2	2	1	11
5	Other pairs	17	15	24	16

	Period of presentation			
	1965–1969	1970–1974	1975–1979	1980–1984
Odds Ratios (Conditional Logistic Regression)	3.0	4.1	10.5	11.6
95% CI	1.0–6.8	0.8–10.5	5.0–153	3.3–72.4

Test for trend: 5.48 (1 df); $P = .0019$.
(Reprinted, with permission, from Wessely et al., 1991.)

ethnicity contribute to the odds ratios (rows 2 and 3). Pairs concordant for ethnicity (rows 1 and 4), or pairs in which either case or control are neither Caucasian nor African-Caribbean (row 5), do not contribute further (Schlesselman, 1982). Odds ratios are therefore the ratio of row 3/ row 2. Confidence intervals were obtained using the formula provided by Gardner and Altman (1989) together with standard tables for the binomial distribution (Neave, 1979).

Conditional logistic regression

Matched case control studies can also be analysed by the more powerful tool of conditional logistic regression, available via the EGRET statistical package. The logistic regression method gives identical odds ratios for the entire study period (i.e. 1964–1984), but the results for each stratum (i.e. 1964–1969; 1970–1974 etc.) are slightly different to those obtained without the aid of the statistical package. This is because logistic regression gives results that are mutually consistent across the study periods, the model in effect "smoothing" both the odds ratios and confidence limits. We present the odds ratios and confidence limits obtained by conditional logistic regression, but have confirmed that the more traditional approaches give similar results for all the analyses presented here, and in particular there is no tendency for either method to report consistently more liberal or conservative results. Each table also includes all the discordant pairs to permit calculation of the conventional odds ratios/confidence limits.

Tests for trends were also obtained using conditional logistic regression. Thus, a possible trend in the risk of schizophrenia in African-Caribbeans over time was assessed by entering an interaction term between ethnicity and period, the resulting likelihood ratio statistic being treated as a chi-squared statistic on one degree of freedom. Again, a test for trend can be calculated directly, using a non-regression method. Because this method uses a continuity correction, the results were generally more conservative (ignoring the continuity correction, as some statisticians advise, would give results very similar to those obtained by regression). Even with the correction, the results differed substantially on only one analysis (Table 9.4), for which both results have been quoted.

Unless otherwise stated, comparisons are made between those of African-Caribbean and Caucasian ethnicity only. However, results are also presented comparing African-Caribbeans with all other groups, thus eliminating row 5 and increasing the power (Tables 9.2, 9.5). For reasons of space only discordant pairs (rows 2 and 3) are presented in Tables 9.3, 9.4, 9.5, 9.6, and 9.7.

Trends in risk, by ethnicity

A total of 130 patients of African-Caribbean ethnicity received a diagnosis of ICD-9 schizophrenia over the two decades. No evidence was found of an ethnicity/gender interaction (see below), so results are presented for both sexes combined. The risk of the illness in African-Caribbeans is increasing across the study period (Table 9.1), particularly between 1964 and 1980. If only cases fulfilling RDC (Table 9.3) or DSM-III–R (Table 9.4) criteria for schizophrenia or schizophreniform psychosis are used, similar trends are seen. That for RDC schizophrenia just fails to reach conventional statistical significance, although this is achieved if the comparison is between African-Caribbeans and all other ethnic groups ($\chi^2 = 6.74$; $P = .009$). The particularly wide confidence limits for the third period reflect the small numbers in Row 2 (pairs in which the case was Caucasian and the control African-Caribbean). Use of 10-year time periods was considered, but, with the exception of Table 9.7 (see below), rejected because of the evidence of period/ethnicity interaction.

TABLE 9.2
ICD Schizophrenia (African-Caribbean Versus all Other Groups)

Matched pair	Period of presentation			
	1965–1969	1970–1974	1975–1979	1980–1984
Case other Control other	83	74	95	74
Case other Control African-Caribbean	8	7	3	4
Case African-Caribbean Control other	16	27	33	38
Case African-Caribbean Control African-Caribbean	2	2	1	11

	Period of presentation			
	1965–1969	1970–1974	1975–1979	1980–1984
Odds Ratios (clr)	2.1	3.8	15.7	9.1
95% CI	0.9–4.7	1.2–11.8	3.0–82.9	2.4–35.0

Test for trend: 7.12; $P = .008$.
(Reprinted, with permission, from Wessely et al., 1991.)

TABLE 9.3
RDC Schizophrenia

Discordant pairs	Period of presentation			
	1965–1969	1970–1974	1975–1979	1980–1984
Case Caucasian Control African-Caribbean	3	4	2	1
Case African-Caribbean Control Caucasian	6	17	24	22

	Period of presentation			
	1965–1969	1970–1974	1975–1979	1980–1984
Odds Ratios (CLR)	2.0	4.2	17.4	33.0
95% CI	0.8–5.3	1.2–18.8	2.4–52.2	3.6 –246.5

Test for trend = 3.32 (1 df); $P = .06$.
(Reprinted, with permission, from Wessely et al., 1991.)

TABLE 9.4
DSM-III–R Schizophrenia And Schizophreniform Disorder

Discordant pairs	Period of presentation			
	1965–1969	1970–1974	1975–1979	1980–1984
Case Caucasian Control African-Caribbean	2	3	2	1
Case African-Caribbean Control Caucasian	6	14	19	17

	Period of presentation			
	1965–1969	1970–1974	1975–1979	1980–1984
Odds Ratios (clr)	1.8	4.7	11.0	18.0
95% CI	0.6–9.0	0.8–31.3	1.4–72.8	1.5–193.0

Test for trend (regression) = 3.56, (df= 1); P = .059.
Test for trend (continuity correction) = 1.86, df= 1; P = .17.
(Reprinted, with permission, from Wessely et al., 1991.)

Analysis of year of birth

When the pairs were analysed by year of birth, rather than year of presentation, there was an increase in risk for later years of birth, most marked for RDC schizophrenia (Table 9.5), and least evident for ICD schizophrenia (χ^2 for trend = -3.08; 1 df; $P < .1 > .5$). Similar results were obtained when comparing only African-Caribbeans and Caucasians (data not shown). This was confirmed by a trend for an interaction between ethnicity and year of birth in the logistic model (likelihood ratio statistic = 3.085; P = .079).

TABLE 9.5
Period Of Birth: RDC Schizophrenia (African-Caribbeans Versus All Other Groups)

	Before 1929	1930–1949	1950–1967
Discordant pairs			
Case other Control African-Caribbean	5	4	3
Case African-Caribbean Control other	8	29	36
Odds Ratios	1.6	7.3	12.0
95% CI	0.3–8.1	1.8–51.5	3.6–38.0

Test for trend = 5.58; df= 1; P = .018.
(Reprinted, with permission, from Wessely et al., 1991.)

First and second generation African-Caribbeans

Table 9.6 shows the risks comparing those of African-Caribbean ethnicity born in the West Indies, with all other groups. Second generation African-Caribbeans now appear along with all other ethnic groups. This has resulted in a substantial fall in the odds ratio for the last time period. Again, the presence of only two cases in row 2 during the third period makes the odds ratios for 1975–1979 unstable. However, comparing the other three time periods suggests that there has not been a marked increase in risk for this group, confirmed by the absence of a significant trend. It was impossible to carry out the same analysis for African-Caribbeans born in the UK because of lack of discordant pairs, even if all time periods were combined. The odds ratio for first generation African-Caribbeans over all other groups was 3.8 (rising to 4.3 if second generation cases were excluded from contributing to other groups). However, although there were 30 second generation African-Caribbean cases, and three second generation controls, all the second generation African-Caribbean controls were paired with second generation cases, so the odds ratio was infinite. However, as the odds ratio could not be less than 10, the data support other findings of a substantial elevation in the risk of schizophrenia in second generation African-Caribbeans.

An alternative was to follow the example of McGovern and Cope (1987), and repeat the analysis with cases and controls including not only those of African-Caribbean ethnicity born in this country, but also those who migrated as children, defined here as before 18 years. Two pairs were eliminated because of lack of information as to when the control entered the UK. Despite widening the definitions, there were still no discordant pairs in the third period. Adjacent quinquennia were therefore combined

TABLE 9.6
Place Of Birth: ICD Schizophrenia (West Indies Versus Elsewhere)

Discordant pairs	1965–1969	1970–1974	1975–1979	1980–1984
Case: Born elsewhere Control: Born West Indies	8	7	2	7
Case: Born West Indies Control: Born elsewhere	19	25	25	23
	1965–1969	1970–1974	1975–1979	1980–1984
Odds Ratios	2.4	3.6	12.0	3.4
95% CI	0.9–4.7	1.1–11.7	2.3–63.7	1.0–11.3

Test for trend = 1.19; $P = .274$
(Reprinted, with permission, from Wessely et al., 1991.)

into two 10-year bands. The results show that the odds ratios increased from 2.6 for 1965–1974, to 8.8 for 1975–1984, although not achieving statistical significance ($\chi^2 = 3.21$; $P < .1 > .05$).

To overcome this problem of lack of power, the sample was simply divided into those born before and after 1955, a year chosen to approximate to the period when second generation children began to be born. Comparing all those of African-Caribbean ethnicity against all other ethnic groups (Table 9.7), the risk of ICD-9 schizophrenia rose after 1955, but only slightly (likelihood ratio statistic = 0.82; $P = .37$). In contrast, comparing those born in the West Indies with all other places of birth, the risk fell after 1955 (likelihood ratio statistic = 3.48; $P = .06$).

The influence of age at migration

The influence of age of entry to the United Kingdom was assessed as follows. Looking only at those born in the West Indies, cases and controls were divided into those who came before age 18, and those who came aged 18 and over. Over the whole time period, the increase in the risk of schizophrenia for those born in the West Indies compared to all other places of birth was 4.1 (95% CI = 2.4–7.3). For those entering aged 18 and above it was 4.9, and those entering at younger ages it was 2.7. For these analyses, African-Caribbeans born in the UK were included with all other places of birth. Excluding them did not alter the odds ratios for those entering as adults, but the risk for those arriving in the UK aged below 18 increased from 2.7 to 3.5.

Gender effects

It has been suggested that the increased risk of schizophrenia in African-Caribbeans is restricted to males (Glover, 1989a), although this has not been a universal finding. The overall odds ratios for the excess of

TABLE 9.7
Influence Of Year Of Entry To UK

	Before 1955	1955 and After
1. African-Caribbean ethnicity versus all other groups	4.5 (2.7–8.0)	7.6 (2.6–22.3)
2. Place of birth West Indies versus all other places of birth	4.8 (2.8–8.1)	1.7 (0.6–4.8)
3. As 2, but excluding all African-Caribbeans born in the UK	4.4 (2.5–8.4)	2.4 (0.8–5.6)

(Reprinted, with permission, from Wessely et al., 1991.)

schizophrenia in African-Caribbean compared to Caucasian males was 9.0 (95% CI = 4.1–19.6), compared to 4.1 (95% CI = 2.1–7.9) for females, a non-significant difference. No interaction was seen between time period and gender ($\chi^2 = 2.35$; $P = .12$).

DISCUSSION

The strategy adopted here avoids some of the methodological problems that have affected previous studies in this area. Uniform diagnostic criteria minimise the effect of changing diagnostic habits over time. Using incident cases eliminates duration bias. Matching for age, sex, and period controls for changes in the age or gender structure of the population.

Our findings are not due to an excess of the so called "brief reactive psychoses". Although it has been suggested that individuals with these conditions are frequently misdiagnosed as schizophrenic in African-Caribbean samples, this has not been confirmed (Harvey et al., 1990). In the current analysis, similar trends were noted when using either RDC (which specifies a minimum period of illness of two weeks) or DSM-III-R criteria for schizophrenia (in which the minimum period of illness is six months).

However, other methodological explanations cannot be excluded. Using operational criteria helps to steer away from the Scylla of idiosyncratic diagnostic habits and cultural biases, but may bring us closer to the Charybdis of committing Kleinman's "category error" (Kleinman, 1977). It is also true that the cross cultural validity of the instruments used has not been specifically established. Nevertheless, we do not feel that such possibilities could explain all our findings, and in particular the time trends. Furthermore, there is no evidence that UK psychiatrists currently overdiagnose schizophrenia in African-Caribbeans (Lewis et al., 1990; McGovern, Hemmings, Cope, & Lowerson, 1994).

A second methodological explanation of these findings is that the age of onset of schizophrenia is differentially decreasing in the African-Caribbean population (Littlewood & Lipsedge, 1988). This would increase the number of cases towards the end of the study period and give a false impression of increasing risk. This explanation cannot be refuted until all the cohort has passed through the period at risk and lifetime morbidity calculated.

A third possibility is that these results are affected by exposure bias. If this was a valid study, then the "exposure" under investigation (ethnicity) would not influence the selection of cases and controls. This assumption may have been violated. Pathways to psychiatric care differ according to ethnic origin (Harrison et al., 1989; Littlewood & Lipsedge, 1982). We have already indicated our belief that the sampling frame reported in these studies is representative of schizophrenia in Camberwell, since nearly all individuals with schizophrenia make contact with the mental health services (Eaton, 1985). However, the controls may not be a representative sample of those with other mental illnesses. It is probable that different biases operate in the way in which non-psychotic individuals of different ethnic groups make contact with services. Some of these biases have been minimised, for example by using all contacts, and not just admission rates. However, others remain. Thus the finding that African-Caribbeans have an increased risk of schizophrenia compared to other mental illnesses, although in keeping with other studies, is subject to bias.

This drawback was reduced by using four sampling periods. All of these are subject to the same bias, but there is little reason to suspect that these biases have changed during the period in question. More robust than the finding of a single elevated risk, is that the risk of schizophrenia in African-Caribbeans is increasing. The use of age-, sex-, and period-matched controls means that this is not due to changes in the age structure or ethnic composition of the Camberwell population. For it to be explained solely on methodological grounds, one must postulate not only a differential effect in the use of mental health services by African-Caribbeans, but one that is declining. There is little support for this in our data. The proportion of African-Caribbean controls rose from 7 to 12% between 1964 and 1984. Between 1961 and 1981, census data show that the proportion of the local population born in the West Indies rose from 2.5% to 6.6%. Thus, the proportion of all African-Caribbeans increased 1.7-fold, compared to a 2.6-fold increase in those born in the Caribbean in the local population. There are no figures for the rate of increase of all African-Caribbeans locally, but in the previous chapter we gave our estimate that in 1981 11.5% of the local population was of African-Caribbean ethnicity. This last figure is very similar to the proportion of African-Caribbean controls in the last time period. In conclusion, there is some evidence that the rate of increase in the number of controls of African-Caribbean ethnicity has not matched that of the local population, but this is not substantial.

Our studies of ethnicity and schizophrenia in Camberwell gave two principal findings. First, that African-Caribbeans are indeed at elevated risk of schizophrenia, and second, that this risk has increased between 1965 and 1980. The latter observation is at variance with reports from various countries of a decline in the incidence of schizophrenia (see Beiser & Iacono, 1990; Der et al., 1990, and discussion in Chapter 8). We have already shown that no such decline has occurred in Camberwell (Chapter 8). This is at least in part due to the high proportion of African-Caribbean residents.

Explanatory hypotheses

We have already discussed the issue of the relationship between different experiences of social adversity, and the differing changes in the incidence of schizophrenia. In contrast to those areas in which schizophrenia has been recorded as declining, such as New Zealand, northeast Scotland, Eire, and Denmark, Camberwell is an area in which indices of social deprivation have worsened during the period in question.

It is beyond dispute that the ethnic minority population of the United Kingdom, and particularly those of African-Caribbean origin, are exposed to wide range of social adversities. Being black is associated with unemployment, inadequate housing, and low social class (Townsend, Phillimore, & Beattie, 1988), as well as disruptions and impairment of family functioning (Brown, 1984). The experience of racism has also been linked to increased rates of mental illness (Littlewood & Lipsedge, 1982). It is probable that any of these factors could directly result in a worse prognosis, and hence higher prevalence, of schizophrenia in the African-Caribbean population.

We argue, in addition, that such factors could affect the incidence of the disease, perhaps by precipitating illness in predisposed individuals. In support of this notion, Jarman and colleagues, using district admission statistics provided by the Mental Health Enquiry, have confirmed that social adversity confounds the relationship between ethnicity and admission to mental hospital. Although being born in the West Indies is significantly associated with mental hospital admission, once adjustment has been made for social deprivation, this association disappears (Jarman, Hirsch, White, & Driscoll, 1992).

Two other studies add further support to the idea that environmental adversity may be related to the differing rates of schizophrenia between African-Caribbean and non-African-Caribbean populations in the UK. Sugarman and Crawford (1994) showed that there were no differences in the morbid risk of developing schizophrenia in the parents of African-Caribbean and Caucasian probands with schizophrenia. Thus, the genetic influences on schizophrenia operated equally in both groups. However, the morbid risk for schizophrenia in the siblings of African-Caribbean subjects with schizophrenia was substantially higher than in Caucasian families. This finding was recently replicated in an independent sample drawn from the Camberwell catchment area; the morbid risk for schizophrenia in the siblings of second generation African-Caribbean schizophrenic patients was approximately six times higher than that in the siblings of white schizophrenics (Hutchinson et al., 1996). This astonishing, but replicated, finding implies the operation of some environmental risk factor on the second generation. The lack of any evidence for a substantial increase in the risk of schizophrenia in the Caribbean itself (Hickling & Rodgers–Johnson, 1995) also argues against genetic explanations of the increased risk of schizophrenia for African-Caribbeans in the UK.

Data from the WHO Determinants of Outcome Study (Jablensky, Sartorius, & Ernberg, 1992) have shown that the prognosis of psychotic disorders such as schizophrenia is better in non-industrialised countries, and some researchers have suggested that African-Caribbeans in the UK might have a similarly good prognosis, and that the increased incidence of psychosis in this group might be due to an excess of good-prognosis illness (Littlewood & Lipsedge, 1981). Follow-up studies to test this hypothesis have not shown a consistently better outcome for African-Caribbeans when compared with British-born Whites or White Europeans (Birchwood et al., 1992; McGovern et al., 1994; Sugarman, 1992). However, this failure may have been due to methodological flaws. Though lower socioeconomic status and early age at onset are related to both ethnic group and poorer outcome (Van Os et al., 1995), the studies have not controlled for these variables. McKenzie and colleagues (1995) compared four-year course and outcome of psychotic illness between African-Caribbean ($n = 53$) and British-born White ($n = 60$) individuals. Participants were patients admitted to two south London hospitals with a recent onset of psychotic illness. The main outcome measures were illness course, self-harm, social disability, hospital use, and treatment variables, and these were adjusted for socio-economic origin, sex, age of onset, and diagnosis. The African-Caribbean group spent more of the follow-up period in a recovered state (adjusted odds ratio (OR) = 5.0), were less likely to have had a continuous, unremitting illness (adjusted OR = 0.3), and were less at risk of self-harm and suicide (adjusted OR = 0.2). There was no evidence for interaction with diagnostic group; on the other hand, they were more likely to be admitted to hospital involuntarily, and more likely to have spent time in jail. In a smaller sample, McGovern et al. (1994) also showed that African-Caribbeans with schizophrenia had increased contact with the forensic and prison services. These results suggest that the high incidence observed in UK African-Caribbeans is coupled with a less deteriorated illness course but one which involves considerable social disruption. An excess of exposure to precipitants in the social environment, resulting in good prognosis "reactive" illness, may be one explanation; an illness onset related to social adversity leads to a good prognosis as regards clinical variables such as symptoms, but a poor prognosis for social outcomes.

Social adversity is not the only possible environmental risk factor which may be operating. Other plausible biological candidates include poor antenatal and perinatal care and infection. Much recent work has suggested that obstetric complications and low birth weight are significantly associated with an increased risk of schizophrenia in offspring (reviewed by Geddes and

Lawrie, 1995). Maternal viral infection during the second trimester of pregnancy has also been associated with schizophrenia in the offspring in studies of the 1957 influenza epidemic, as well as other influenza epidemics (reviewed by McGrath & Castle, 1995).

Both these factors could be more marked in the African-Caribbean population in the UK. Maternal death rates are 10 times higher in Jamaica than in England (Walker, Ashley, McCaw, & Bernard, 1986). It is also known that UK-born African-Caribbean babies have lower birth weights than either Caucasian or Asian infants, yet paradoxically rates of perinatal mortality are also lower (Pearson, 1991; Terry, Condie, Bissenden, & Kerridge, 1987). Thus, an increase in the number of low birth weight infants surviving to adulthood could, in theory, be a factor underlying the high rates of schizophrenia in second generation African-Caribbeans. However, in contrast it must also be pointed out that children born in the UK to mothers from the Caribbean have unusually low rates of stillbirth and perinatal mortality due to congenital and central nervous system abnormalities (Balarajan, Raleigh, & Botting, 1989). Furthermore, Hutchinson et al. (1996) have recently compared the frequency of obstetric complications in White and African-Caribbean psychotic patients seen at the Maudsley Hospital; obstetric complications were almost twice as common in the White patients. Other indirect evidence against obstetric complications playing an important causal role in the excess of schizophrenia in the African-Caribbean population arises from the evidence that individuals with schizophrenia who have a history of obstetric complications or low birth weight tend to have more developmental problems in childhood than those without such a history (Rifkin et al., 1994). McKenzie et al. (1995) have found that African-Caribbean schizophrenia patients were less likely to have had neurodevelopmental or neurological problems in childhood than their white counterparts.

Prenatal viral exposure cannot be excluded by retrospective maternal interview, and therefore remains a possible factor. Individuals brought up in the Caribbean are more likely to be seronegative to certain viruses such as rubella, since even in Jamaica the population is too small to maintain endemic rubella, and there was no schoolgirl immunisation programme until 1978. As many young women migrated to the United Kingdom during the 1950s, first generation African-Caribbean mothers were highly susceptible to rubella (see Nicoll & Logan, 1989), which explains high rates of congenital rubella in their children (Parsons, 1983). A similar model has been proposed to explain increased rates of severe mental retardation in the offspring of African-Caribbean women recently arrived in this country (Wing, 1979). It is thus possible that another consequence of maternal exposure to viral illness, whether in the West Indies or United Kingdom, is an increased risk of adult schizophrenia (Glover, 1989b; Harrison, 1990).

Such exposures may also change over time. Glover (1989a) used hospital admission data for two London regions to show that the increased risk of schizophrenia is most marked in males born in the Caribbean after 1950, and has proposed that these results reflect a cohort effect. It is possible that such an effect may be a result of epidemics during the same period, analogous to the effects of influenza epidemics. During the 1950s the Caribbean suffered a number of infectious epidemics; for example, epidemic poliomyelitis only arrived in Jamaica in 1954 (Luck, 1966). We found that for those born in the West Indies, a peak was reached by the early 1950s, and fell subsequently. At least part of this increase will be an artifact of emigration, since a proportion of those predisposed to develop schizophrenia may have become ill in the Caribbean, and thus not emigrated. This would differentially affect the older birth cohorts. Nevertheless, the data partially support a cohort effect for young men born in the Caribbean between 1950 and 1960 as suggested by previous work (Glover, 1989a).

However, if one postulates exposure to an infective factor, then our results suggest increased maternal exposure to infection not only before migration, but also after. Furthermore, maternal exposure to unfamiliar viruses has much less explanatory power when related to the increase in the risk of schizophrenia seen in those of African origin (see Chapter 10).

A high prevalence of cannabis abuse has put forward by some as another explanation for the high rate of schizophrenia in African-Caribbeans in the UK. However, the role of cannabis in causing schizophrenia in those without underlying predisposition remains controversial (see Castle & Ames, 1996). Furthermore, McGuire et al. (1995) reported no significant difference in the frequency with which cannabis was found in the urine of African-Caribbean and White psychotic patients admitted to hospitals in south London. A further argument against an explanation on the basis of differential consumption comes from Holland. Selten and Sijben (1994) have shown that migrants to The Netherlands from the Caribbean also have an increased incidence of schizophrenia; however, they have a lower consumption of cannabis than the native Dutch population.

CONCLUSION

Reviewing the Camberwell Register studies in the context of other studies of ethnicity and schizophrenia confirms that there has been a true increase in the risk of schizophrenia in African-Caribbeans resident in the UK. The balance of evidence points to environmental factors affecting the risk of schizophrenia that continue to operate at all ages. We suggest that several factors may be responsible for the increasing risk of schizophrenia in

African-Caribbeans, and that these factors may operate at various periods, both prenatally and in adult life. All these factors may in turn be related to social adversity and deprivation. Schizophrenia researchers may observe that attention must continue to be paid to social factors in the aetiology of schizophrenia. Others may conclude that as long as ethnicity and social adversity remain closely correlated, separating out the various effects will be difficult. Extension of these analyses, to encompass the more accurate demographic data from the 1991 Census, is presented in Chapter 10.

CHAPTER TEN

Psychotic illness in ethnic minorities: Evidence from the 1991 UK Census

We have shown in Chapter 8 that the first-contact incidence of schizophrenia and mania did not decrease in Camberwell over the period 1965–84, and that the likely reason for the discrepancy between this and previous studies which had demonstrated a decline in first-contact rates lay in the changes in the ethnic composition of the source population over the period under investigation. Harrison (1990) has reviewed incidence studies of schizophrenia amongst African-Caribbean migrants to the UK, and concluded that rates of this disorder are high amongst such individuals. We have also shown that the excess in Camberwell is not due to misdiagnosis (see also Harrison et al., 1988; Lewis et al., 1990; and Chapter 9), or to admission bias, as our results were similar regardless of whether we selected first-contact cases or first admission cases (see also Bebbington et al., 1981; Harrison et al., 1988). Although much of the current focus has been on schizophrenia in the African-Caribbean population, we have shown in Chapter 8 that the excess is not specific to schizophrenia (see also Leff et al., 1976; Harrison et al., 1988), and an early study suggests that high rates may not be specific to the African-Caribbean population (Rwegellera, 1977).

The case–control study reported in Chapter 9 lends further support to the view that the African-Caribbean population in the UK is at increased risk of schizophrenia. However, valid epidemiological evidence has been lacking, because of the absence of reliable figures on the size and age structure of ethnic minority populations; this has been a source of much criticism (Burke, 1989; Jablensky, 1993; Sashidharan, 1993).

125

The 1991 Census was the first in England and Wales to include comprehensive data on the ethnic composition of the general population, providing a unique opportunity to assess accurately the incidence of both schizophrenia and other psychoses in not only African-Caribbean and white groups, but also in other ethnic comparison groups. One recent study (King et al., 1994) used census figures to calculate the first-contact incidence of schizophrenia in ethnic minorities over a one-year period. The results suggested that membership of any ethnic minority group was a risk factor for psychosis, but numbers were too small to draw conclusions for individual ethnic groups.

We therefore now proceed to investigate first-admission rates for operationally defined schizophrenia and related conditions in Camberwell over the period of 1985–1992, employing the 1991 Census data to establish denominators for African-Caribbean and white groups. As there has also been a recent increase in the number of Africans living in Camberwell, we were able also to examine rates for Africans; together these three groups constitute more than 90% of the population in the area.

THE CURRENT STUDY

For this study, we had to extend our analyses beyond the period of functioning of the Camberwell Register, to ascertain more recent trends in the incidence of the disorders under study, as well as to utilise the contemporary denominator data provided by the 1991 general population census. As noted above, the 1991 Census was the first in England and Wales to include information about ethnicity, thus allowing us to assess the possible influence of changing ethnic composition of the general population, on rates of psychosis. Data are presented in full in Van Os et al. (1996a).

The difficulty in extending the analyses to 1992 lie in the Camberwell Register having ceased to function in 1984, forcing us to rely on admission data alone for the period 1985 to 1992, as indicated in Chapter 2. We were encouraged that this method was suitable by the findings, reported in Chapter 3, of no significant change over the period 1965 to 1984 in the proportion of patients actually being admitted at first contact with the psychiatric services, as well as the lack of any ethnic bias in admission policies over this period. There is no reason to suspect that these trends would have changed for the period 1985 to 1992, as psychiatric service provision for the Camberwell changed little over this time.

However, we did find, as is detailed in Chapter 3, that there were systematic differences in illness characteristics and sociodemographic variables between admitted and non-admitted patients, and thus restricted the use of the 1985–1992 data only for those analyses for which they were essential; that is, for assessing ethnic influences.

We had to devise as close a match as possible of the case finding for the years 1985–1992, for the 20 years of case finding covered by the Register itself. To this end, a list was generated from the Maudsley/ Bethlem Royal Hospitals computerised admission index of all first-admission patients from the Camberwell area (defined as exactly the same geographical area as that from which the Camberwell Register drew its patients), who had their first admission during the period, and who received a discharge diagnosis of "schizophrenia" and related conditions (including "schizoaffective disorder"; ICD-9 codes 295.0–295.9), paraphrenia (297.2), or "other non-organic psychoses" (298.1–298.9). Again, the broad sample was chosen so as to reduce the possibility of missing any patients who had been inappropriately labelled, and to allow for diagnostic trends. By the period 1985–1992, the Maudsley/Bethlem Royal Hospitals had become responsible for providing all National Health Service psychiatric care for people living in Camberwell. Unfortunately, the hospitals recorded only diagnostic data on patients admitted, not all contacts.

For those patients admitted to the Maudsley/Bethlem Royal Hospitals between 1985 and 1992, DJC, JVO, and another psychiatrist colleague (Dr Nori Takei, Senior Lecturer, Department of Psychological Medicine, Institute of Psychiatry, UK) rated around a third of the cases each, using OCCPI 2.5, as for the Camberwell Register patients themselves (see Chapter 2). For the analyses relating to this period, we used exclusively RDC diagnoses, for which an independent reliability exercise resulted in a mean kappa for the three raters of 0.74.

Over the period 1985–1992, a total of 167 patients with first contact, first-admission non-affective, non-organic psychosis were identified; case records could be located for all patients but two. One hundred and nineteen patients fulfilled RDC diagnostic criteria for schizophrenia.

Demographic data concerning the general population of Camberwell were supplied by the Office of Population Censuses and Surveys (OPCS). Data from the 1991 Census (100% sample) were used, and population estimates for the previous and subsequent years (1988–1990, 1992) were interpolated. There are a number of problems with the Census, which are unlikely to be fully resolved by the Census Validation Survey. We therefore attempted to adjust for these in a conservative manner, i.e. biased towards the null hypothesis of no differences in rates of schizophrenia between the white and other ethnic groups. Ethnic groups in the Census include a sizeable group "other Blacks", which comprises both African-Caribbean, African, and other individuals (e.g. "Black British"). As it was not possible to further divide this group, it was added in its entirety to both the African-Caribbean and African populations in the denominator for the calculation of rates.

A second issue is that of sex-related underenumeration among the younger age groups in the Census. Although females outnumbered males in all three ethnic groups under investigation, the ratio of males to females in the population aged between 15 and 44 years was 0.94 for the white group, 0.87 for the African group, and 0.69 for the African-Caribbean group. A simple correction was therefore made, such that the number of African-Caribbean and African males in the age group 15 to 44 was increased to yield a sex ratio of unity (effectively increasing the denominator in the age groups most at risk for schizophrenia, and thus reducing rates for schizophrenia; see Table 10.1).

According to Siegel (1974), underreporting in the US census may be in the region of 4 to 18% in black men, compared to 1 to 4% in white men. There is anecdotal evidence of a similar ethnic discrepancy in the 1991 British census. We therefore applied, in addition to the above adjustments, a general 20% underreporting correction for the African-Caribbean and African groups, which again would tend to decrease incidence rates (Table 10.1).

Five-year rates for RDC schizophrenia and other psychosis were calculated, based on the census figures for the population at risk in Camberwell, i.e. those aged 16 years and over. Unadjusted rates were

TABLE 10.1

Example Of Correction For Gender-Related And General Under-Enumeration In The 1991 Census, Shown For The Group African-Caribbean Males And "Other Black" Males In Camberwell

	African-Caribbean and "Other Black" Groups		
	A	B	C
Age Group	Census Figures*	Correction 1*	Correction 2 (B*100/80)
0–14	2514	2514	3143
15–24	1361	1589	1986
25–34	1523	2383	2979
35–44	580	1002	1253
45–54	794	794	993
55–64	933	933	1166
65–74	350	350	438
75+	54	54	68
Total	8109	9619	12026

* Underlined figures point towards a discrepancy in the gender distribution, and subsequent corrections, which consisted of an increase of the number of males in the age-groups 15–44, such that the sex ratio in these age groups was unity (see text).

(From Van Os et al., 1996a. Reprinted with the permission of Cambridge University Press.)

compared using the rate ratio (RR). Indirect standardisation was used to adjust for age and sex: the expected number of cases in each stratum of the study population (ethnic minority groups) was calculated by multiplying the stratum-specific rates of the standard population (white population) by the number of person-years of the study population in that category; differences in adjusted rates were expressed as the standard mortality ratio (SMR). The SMR can, similar to the incidence rate ratio, be interpreted as the ratio of incidences in the exposed and the non-exposed group; the SMR was used here because the method of indirect standardisation can better cope with small numbers of cases in the age- and sex-specific strata. Three broad age bands were used (16–34, 35–54, 55+). Exact confidence limits were calculated where the observed number of cases (d) was less than 10; for d10 approximate confidence intervals are given (Breslow & Day, 1987; Rothman, 1986).

Rates for first-contact, first-admission schizophrenia

A total of 110 patients with first-contact, first-admission non-affective psychosis were identified; case records could be located for all of them, and 79 fulfilled RDC diagnostic criteria for schizophrenia (Table 10.2). The remaining 31 patients were labelled "other psychosis". There were no significant differences in the proportion of patients receiving a schizophrenic diagnosis in the different ethnic groups ($\chi^2 = 0.1$; 3 df; $P = .9$). The distribution of cases over the five consecutive years was rather similar in the main ethnic groups: white group: 12,11,8,11,2; African-Caribbean group: 4,8,10,6,1; African group: 9,6,6,8,3.

The total five-year incidence of schizophrenia, using unadjusted census figures, was 79 per 515,626 person-years, yielding a five-year rate of 15.3

TABLE 10.2
Diagnostic Distribution Of First-Contact, First-Admission Cases Of Non-Affective Psychosis By Ethnicity, Camberwell 1988–1992

Ethnic group	ICD non-affective psychosis*	RDC schizophrenia (%)
White	44	30 (68%)
African-Caribbean	29	22 (76%)
African	32	23 (72%)
Other	5	4 (80%)
Total	110	79 (72%)

* Includes ICD "schizophrenic psychoses" (295.0–295.9), "paraphrenia" (297.2), and "other non-organic psychoses" (298.1–298.9).

(From Van Os et al., 1996a. Reprinted with the permission of Cambridge University Press.)

per 100,000 person-years (95% CI = 12.3–19.1). The number of schizophrenic individuals of "other ethnicity" ($n = 4$) was deemed too small and heterogeneous to yield meaningful measures of effect, and were not included in the comparative analyses. Rates for schizophrenia, unadjusted for sex, age and underenumeration were: (1) white group: 7.8 per 100,000 person-years (95% CI = 5.4–11.1); (2) African-Caribbean group: 34.4 per 100,000 person-years (95% CI = 22.6–52.3); (3) African group: 53.2 per 100,000 person-years (95% CI = 35.5–80.1), yielding unadjusted rate ratios of 4.4 (2.4–7.3) and 6.8 (4.3–10.9), respectively. Adjusting for age, gender and underenumeration yielded SMRs of 3.1 (2.0–4.7) and 4.2 (2.8–6.2) respectively (Table 10.3). Thus, adjustment for age, sex and underenumeration reduced both measures of effect by 30–40%. The SMRs for RDC schizophrenia were high both in the age group 16–34 years, as well as in the group aged 35 to 54 years, although the confidence intervals in the latter were wider due to the small number of subjects (Table 10.3). We also compared rates of "other psychosis", adjusting for age, sex and underenumeration as described above. The SMR for the African-Caribbean and African groups combined (in view of the small numbers) versus the white group was 2.4 (1.4–3.8).

DISCUSSION

Standardised rates for operationalised schizophrenia were higher not only in the African-Caribbean group, but also in the African group, after correction for age- and gender-related underreporting in the census data, and a 20% underestimate of the size of the African-Caribbean and African populations.

Methodological issues

Our rates represent, of course, an underestimate of the real incidence of schizophrenia, as we selected cases on the basis of admission to hospital only. However, the unadjusted rate of 1.5 per 10,000 person-years is close to that reported by Cooper and colleagues (1987). Furthermore, the main focus was on between-group differences in rates and, as detailed in Chapter 3, it is unlikely that an ethnic bias in admission policy has contributed significantly to the results. Although we cannot exclude differential pathways to care for the white group and other ethnic groups, it is unlikely that any pathway bias would have lead to spurious results, because the great majority of incident cases of schizophrenia are eventually admitted to hospital (Cooper et al., 1987).

Although it has been claimed that it is unlikely that there are ethnic biases in rates of underenumeration (Teague, 1993), that conclusion was

TABLE 10.3

Age-Specific, Sex-Adjusted And Age-Adjusted SMR For First-Admission, First-Contact Schizophrenia By Ethnicity, 1988–1992, After Correction For Estimates Of Age- And Gender-Related Underreporting In The Census And A 20% Underestimate Of The Size Of The African-Caribbean And African Populations*

Rate RDC schizophrenia

Age group	White group	African-Caribbean group			African group		
	Observed cases	Observed cases	Expected cases	SMR	Observed cases	Expected cases	SMR
16–34	18	18	6.0	3.0 (1.9–4.8)	22	5.0	4.4 (2.9–6.6)
35–54	3	3	0.6	5.0 (1.01–14.4)	1	0.4	2.5 (0.1–14.2)
55+	9	1	0.6	1.7 (0.1–10.2)	0	0.1	0
16–55+	30	22	7.2	3.1 (2.0–4.7)	23	5.5	4.2 (2.8–6.2)

* Includes the whole category "other blacks".

(From Van Os et al., 1996a. Reprinted with the permission of Cambridge University Press.)

based on a comparison with Labour Force Surveys, which are likely to show the same ethnic biases as the census (Burke, 1989). As we have shown, underenumeration of ethnic minorities is likely to be a real problem in inner city areas, especially as those missing are in the age range most at risk for schizophrenia. Therefore, epidemiological studies should introduce at least a 10%–20% correction for differential underenumeration.

Ethnicity for cases was not ascertained in the same manner as for the population used in the denominator, as in the latter self-reporting in response to census questions about ethnicity was the source of information. Such a numerator–denominator bias could lead to an underestimation of the size of the ethnic minority populations in relation to the cases in the numerator. We have demonstrated, however, that our results are quite robust to possible underenumeration. Furthermore, inclusion of the entire "other black" group will have minimised this problem. The investigators were not blind to ethnicity in rating the OCCPI checklist, but diagnosis was made "blind" by a computer programme. Furthermore, rates were high in ethnic minority groups regardless of diagnosis.

In a previous study in the same area, we reported an association between onset of schizophrenia and lower social class (Castle et al., 1993). Social class may therefore have confounded our results. We were not able to adjust for socioeconomic status as we did not have access to age by sex by class by ethnicity census data. A 10% census sample, however, showed that African-Caribbean economically active residents aged 16 and over in Camberwell were 1.8 (95% CI = 1.7–1.9) times more likely to be unemployed than their white counterparts and 2.1 (95% CI = 1.7–2.6) times more likely to belong to social classes IV and V. For the African group, the odds were 2.2 (2.1–2.4) and 2.5 (1.9–3.3), respectively. Although suggestive, these differences are small compared to the reported SMRs of schizophrenia; if social class were to account for the whole difference in rates between the white and black groups, the effect size of class would need to be around 4–5 times greater that the SMR (Rothman, 1986).

The numbers of schizophrenia cases in the ethnic minority groups may have been exaggerated by the effect of large numbers of young vulnerable ethnic minority individuals drifting into deprived inner city areas with a more stable (and healthy) white population. This factor may especially apply to African migrants, who, compared to the African-Caribbean population, have a less stable population base in Camberwell. However, in both ethnic minority groups, first admission rates were elevated also in the older age group of 35 to 54 year olds, which makes it unlikely that differential mobility has significantly contributed to the results.

Accepting the limitations arising out of the inability to control satisfactorily for socioeconomic status and differential mobility, and the different methods used to ascertain ethnicity for cases and for the general population, the results do support the notion of higher incidence rates of schizophrenia among the African-Caribbean and African populations in Camberwell, the "true" rate ratios, compared to the white group, lying between 2.0–4.7 and 2.8–6.2, respectively.

Several British studies have reported high rates of mental illness in a variety of ethnic minority groups (Rwegellera, 1977; King et al., 1994). These data are also compatible with that from other European countries which show an increased incidence of both affective and non-affective psychosis in migrants and their offspring from the Caribbean and Morocco (Harrison, 1990; King et al., 1994; Selten & Sijben, 1994; Van Os et al., 1996a,d). It would appear that ethnic group as a risk factor for severe mental disorder is not diagnosis specific; risk estimates vary between two and five times for both RDC mania and RDC schizophrenia and other psychoses.

These findings have important implications for various specific explanatory hypotheses for the excess of psychotic disorders amongst African-Caribbeans in the UK, such as the use of cannabis (McGovern & Cope, 1987) and biological theories (Eagles, 1991; Wessely et al., 1991). Whilst these factors may play a role, a non-specific increase in psychosis among various ethnic minority groups would appear to indicate that common sources of stress on members of ethnic minorities, such as cultural adjustment, discrimination, impact of migration and racism, may also be important determinants. Such factors warrant further systematic investigation.

CHAPTER ELEVEN

The longitudinal perspective: The Camberwell collaborative psychosis study

Historically, the schizophrenia concept is defined not only in terms of symptoms in the acute phase, but also of the course. Thus, the Case Register findings reported in this book also need to be viewed from a longitudinal perspective. To facilitate this, we used data from a four-year follow-up of patients with a recent onset psychotic illness, ascertained over the years 1986–1989 (the Camberwell Collaborative Psychosis Sample). In particular, we focus on gender, psychopathology, and ethnic group, to complement and expand our findings from the previous chapters. In addition, we examine the issues of heterogeneity of risk factors and classification of psychosis that were addressed in Chapter 1, from a longitudinal perspective.

THE CURRENT STUDY

The Camberwell Collaborative Psychosis sample was selected from a survey of all admissions for psychosis to the Maudsley, Bethlem Royal, and King's College hospitals from March 1986–February 1988 and October 1988–August 1989 (Harvey et al., 1990; Jones et al., 1993). In order to limit the eligible patients to a number manageable by two interviewers, admissions from each hospital were excluded every third month in rotation. All patients were assessed for inclusion within three days of admission. Inclusion criteria were: age 16–60 years and presence of delusions, hallucinations, or formal thought disorder, as defined by the Research Diagnostic Criteria, in clear consciousness.

Patients whose illness had started within five years of recruitment were selected for the four-year follow-up study ($n = 191$). Thus, a sample was obtained of relatively recent onset of illness, minimising the fallacy of mixing follow-up epochs, which has a potential confounding effect (McGlashan, 1986).

Baseline assessments

Baseline assessments were generally completed within three days of admission. Socioeconomic status at birth or during early childhood was assessed using the Registrar General's classification of paternal occupation. Marital status and employment status were also assessed.

Individuals who had used *illegal substances* more than once in the month before baseline assessment, or alcohol in excess of 50 standard units per week, were classified as "misusing alcohol or drugs".

Information on *obstetric complications* (OCs) was obtained through maternal interview by a rater who was blind to proband characteristics. OCs were rated as absent or definitively present according to the scale of Lewis, Owen, and Murray (1989), except that rapid labour was no longer classified as an OC. This scale had been previously validated by O'Callaghan, Larkin, and Waddington (1990).

Place of birth and place of parents' birth were used as proxy variables to define different *ethnic groups*. Patients were asked their place of birth and their parents' place of birth. Those patients who were white skinned, who were born in the UK, and whose parents were born in the UK comprised the White British group; those who had both parents born in the Caribbean constituted the African-Caribbean group.

Age at onset was defined as appearance of first symptoms of psychosis, and duration of illness was defined as the difference between age at onset, and age at index assessment.

Premorbid adjustment was measured with the Philips scale social adjustment section (1953), based on maternal interviews, conducted by a rater who was blind to the proband's characteristics including diagnosis. The Philips scale is a simple seven-point ordered categorical scale.

Psychopathology was measured using the Present State Examination (Wing et al., 1974), conducted by three experienced clinicians who had received PSE training at the same centre. The Operational Criteria Checklist for Psychotic Illness (OCCPI; McGuffin et al., 1991) was also completed for all patients for the time up to index assessment, to give index diagnoses. Psychopathological data were derived from detailed cross-sectional mental states at index assessment, on the basis of the PSE, and from the patients' case records. Thus, psychopathology ratings used in the analyses (see below) were derived from both cross-sectional interview and more longitudinal case note assessments (Brockington et al., 1992).

Symptom dimensions were identified by extracting initial unrotated factors with principal component analysis on the correlation matrix of the OCCPI checklist, reduced to 20 main items. Factors with an eigenvalue greater than 1 were then subjected to varimax rotation. Finally, regression factor scores were produced for each case for subsequent analyses. Factor loadings smaller than 0.5 were omitted. Thus, a comprehensive list of affective and psychotic symptoms and signs remained, including age of onset and type of onset. Manic and depressive symptoms were each entered as the sum of the ratings on the individual items for mania and depression.

The factor analysis of the 20 OCCPI items yielded a pattern of segregation onto 7 factors, explaining 63% of the variance. The first factor had heavy loadings for bizarre behaviour, catatonia, inappropriate affect, and difficult rapport; the second for bizarre delusions, passivity phenomena, thought interference, and hallucinations; the third for mania, grandiose delusions, and relation between affective and psychotic symptoms; the fourth for early and insidious onset, and blunting of affect; the fifth for symptoms of depression and depressive delusions; the sixth for lack of insight; and the seventh for paranoid delusions (mainly persecutory delusions and delusions of reference). These factors were designated, respectively, inappropriate–catatonia, delusions–hallucinations, mania, insidious–blunting, depression, lack of insight, and paranoid delusions.

CT scanning. This method is described in detail elsewhere (Jones et al., 1994b). Axial CT scans were all performed on a Siemens 9800 Scanner. Slices 1cm thick, parallel to the floor of the anterior fossa and ascending to the vertex were analysed at an independent video console (IVC). Three raters, blind to other information on the proband, each rated an equal proportion of cases. Interrater reliability was assessed using around 100 measures by each rater, obtained from a sample of 10 patients (i.e. 10 structures were measured in each patient).

Family history. Information on psychiatric history of first-degree relatives was obtained from three sources: (1) the proband's medical records; (2) the proband's mother using the FH-RDC; and (3) the medical records of relatives with a psychiatric history. Two familial loading scores for psychiatric disorder were calculated for each proband. First, a familial loading score for schizophrenia was calculated. Second, a familial loading score for affective disorders was calculated. A narrow definition of family history of affective disorder was used (owing to the common and non-specific nature of broadly defined depression), including only relatives with a diagnosis of bipolar disorder or with a diagnosis of major depression requiring psychiatric admission.

Life events. The recording and rating of life events has been described in detail elsewhere (Bebbington et al., 1993). Briefly, individuals with a datable onset of psychotic symptoms were interviewed for a history of events during the six months prior to onset, rated according to the "contextual rating of threat" technique developed by Brown and Harris (1978). Datable onset was defined as an abrupt change, with the emergence of florid symptoms (see Van Os et al., 1994). All non-datable onsets were classified as "insidious". Events were rated along a four-point scale, a rating of 1 indicating "marked threat", 2 "moderate threat", 3 "mild threat", and 4 "no threat". In practice, events were analysed mainly by using a category combining the ratings "1" and "2", and a category containing events rated "3", the main role of events rated "4" being to allow the event history to be overinclusive. A second rating was of the degree to which the event was apparently imposed upon patients and could not be regarded as arising from symptomatic behaviour; events were thus divided into those that are "logically independent", "possibly independent", and "probably dependent". In the baseline life event study, we found the greatest discrepancy between cases and community controls for the more severe events (i.e. rating 1 or 2) in the combined category of independent and possibly independent events in the three months immediately prior to onset. In the present study, therefore, a history was considered positive for stressful events if a person had experienced this type of event prior to onset of illness.

Follow-up assessments

Follow-up data were collected by a psychiatrist, blind to all index data, except sex and ethnic group. Multiple sources of information were used for the follow-up assessments and, where possible and with the patient's permission, general practitioners, family members, spouses, hospital and hostel staff, and case records were consulted (median number of informants: 2; range: 0–3). Instruments used were the Iager scale for the assessment of negative symptoms (Iager, Kirch, & Wyatt, 1985), the WHO Disability Assessment Schedule (Jablensky, Schwartz, & Tomov, 1980), and the Hamilton Depression Rating Scale (Hamilton, 1960). We also used a modified version of the WHO life chart (WHO, 1993), which assesses longitudinally employment, independent living, and hospitalisation, self-harm, and treatments received; it also assesses severity of illness course, using clear definitions for all ratings.

In the analyses regarding ethnic group, data on five areas of treatment over the follow-up were additionally collected. These areas of treatment were: time on antipsychotics, and whether the patient had had anti-depressants, mood stabilising medication, psychotherapy, rehabilitation, or an admission under a section of the Mental Health Act over the follow-up period.

To test the hypothesis that outcome of psychiatric illness is a multidimensional construct (Strauss & Carpenter, 1978), a factor analysis was conducted of all 21 outcome ratings to identify different clinical and social outcome domains (Van Os et al., 1996b). The domains identified were: (1) negative symptoms/social disability; (2) severity of illness course; (3) time living independently; (4) unemployment; (5) imprisonment and vagrancy; and (6) depression/self-harm. Rather than calculating factor scores for each domain, the meaning of which is difficult to appreciate in relation to clinical practice, 13 *a priori* chosen outcome measures were identified (Van Os et al., 1996b).

Course type was rated as "continuous" (no remission longer than six months), "neither episodic nor continuous", "episodic" (no episode longer than six months), and "not psychotic" in this period. A "usual severity of symptoms" rating indicates the symptomatic level of the patient during most of the follow-up period; ratings were "severe", "moderate", "mild" or "recovered". Self-harm included all attempts at self-harm, regardless of the outcome (i.e. both parasuicide and completed suicide were included).

Outcome and predictor measures

A summary of outcome measures is provided in Table 11.1; a summary of the predictors is provided in Table 11.2. The number of cases examined with each predictor is also depicted. These numbers varied because not all individuals had undergone all predictor assessments at baseline. For example, life events could only be measured in patients who had a datable onset, and not all patients consented to CT scanning. There was no evidence for large or significant differences on important baseline variables (age, sex, class, ethnic group, diagnosis) between cases who did and cases who did not have predictor assessments.

Analyses

The measures of course and outcome were the dependent variables, while the various putative predictors of course and outcome (sex, ethnic group, life events, familial morbid risk, premorbid adjustment, cerebral ventricle size, symptom dimensions) served as the independent "exposures". The means of continuous variables, and the proportions for binary variables were compared between the various exposure groups. Means were adjusted

TABLE 11.1
Dimensions Of Course And Outcome, Mean Sample Values, And Scales Used To
Cover These

Dimension of course	Variable used	Mean/proportion‡ (95% CI§)
Negative symptoms/ disability	Mean Iager scale weighted score (range 0–3.9†)	1.69 (1.54–1.75)
	Mean DAS-score* (range 0–4.8†)	1.90 (1.77–2.10)
	Negative symptoms usually present	50% (42%–59%)
Illness severity	Usual symptom severity "recovered"	49% (40%–57%)
	Non-remitting course of illness	44% (35%–52%)
Time living independently	Mean time in hospital	9.3% (7.6%–11.2%)
	Mean time living independently	77.1% (66.9%–77.3%)
Unemployment	Mean time unemployed	51.7% (45.7%–57.7%)
	Employed at follow-up	32% (24%–40%)
Imprisonment/ vagrancy	Imprisonment	15% (10%–22%)
	Vagrancy	6% (3%–11%)
Depression/self-harm	Self-harm/suicide	20% (14%–28%)
	Mean HAMD-score (range: 0–22†)	3.4 (2.9–4.0)

* Disability assessment schedule.
† Higher scores indicate greater severity.
‡ Continuous variables: mean (geometric mean for log-transformed distributions); binary variables: proportions.
§ Exact confidence intervals.

using multiple regression, and proportions using logistic regression, yielding odds ratios. Variables measuring time (time spent in hospital, time unemployed, etc.), were expressed as the proportion of the length of the individual follow-up period. Skewed variables that inclined towards two clinically meaningful categories were dichotomized using the modal value as the cut-off; for example, course of illness was transformed into "continuous" (continuous) and "non-continuous" (neither episodic nor continuous, episodic, and not psychotic), and usual symptom severity into "recovered" (recovered) and "non-recovered" (mild, moderate, and severe).

For all the predictor assessments, relevant confounding factors were identified and adjusted for. A list of the confounders adjusted for is given in Table 11.2.

RESULTS

Of the 191 patients who met inclusion criteria, adequate follow-up data were obtained on 166 (87%) over a period of 18 months. Seven patients had committed suicide, and two had died of other causes. One hundred

TABLE 11.2
Predictors Of Course And Outcome, And Relevant Confounding Factors Adjusted For
In The Analyses

Predictor	Number of cases	Adjustment for:
Sex		See Fig. 1
Men	107	
Women	59	
Ethnic group		Social class, sex, age of onset,
African–Caribbean	53	diagnosis
British White	60	
Life events (LE)		Sex, ethnic group, diagnosis
LE +	30	
LE −	29	
Family history		Diagnosis, age of onset, sex,
Schizophrenia score	150	ethnic group, duration of illness
Affective disorder score	150	
Premorbid adjustment		Sex, age, age of onset, duration of
Philips' scale score	149	illness, diagnosis
Cerebral ventricle size		Sex, age, diagnosis, ethnic group,
Sylvian fissures volume	140	social class, head size, duration
Lateral ventricle volume	140	of illness
Third ventricle volume	140	
Psychopathology		Sex, marital status, premorbid
Insidious–blunting score	166	adjustment
Delusions–hallucinations score	166	
Inappropriate–catatonia score	166	
Mania score	166	
Depression score	166	
Other delusions score	166	
Lack of insight score	166	

fifty-three patients were interviewed personally, four over the telephone, and of the patients not interviewed, high-quality information was available on a further thirteen. Compared to the 166 follow-up patients, the 25 patients not followed up were very similar in age, sex, ethnicity, index diagnosis, paternal social class, and age and type of onset. Thus, it is unlikely that any bias was introduced due to differential attrition.

Cohort characteristics

Of the 166 follow-up patients, 59 (36%) were female, and the mean age at baseline assessment was 26.4 years (range = 16–50; SD = 6.5). At baseline assessment, 88 (53%) had a DSM-III-R diagnosis of schizophrenia or schizophreniform disorder, 43 (26%) of affective psychosis (depressive and bipolar psychoses), 12 (7%) of schizoaffective psychosis, and 23 (14%) of delusional disorder or unspecified functional psychosis. White Europeans comprised 53% of the cohort, and 60 of these had both parents born in the UK.

The mean duration of illness prior to baseline assessment was 2.2 years (SD = 2.0); 70 patients (42%) were first admissions. There were no significant differences in duration of illness between males and females (range of means: 2.0–2.2), ethnic groups (range of means: 2.0–2.5), or social classes (range of means: 1.8–2.4), nor in age of onset of first psychotic symptoms between the ethnic ($F = 0.6$; $P = .6$) and social groups ($F = 0.002$; $P = 1.0$). Males and females showed the expected (Castle & Murray, 1991) difference in age of onset (males: 22.7 years; females: 25.2 years; $t = -2.3$; $P = .03$). Similarly, the mean age of onset was highest for the affective psychoses (25.9 years), and lowest for schizophrenia (21.7 years), with schizoaffective and other psychoses in between (23.2 and 24.9 respectively).

Predictors

The results regarding the effect of the predictors are summarised in Table 11.3. Associations are presented in terms of the direction of statistically significant effects (for details regarding exact effect sizes, please see McKenzie et al., 1995; Navarro, Van Os, Jones, & Murray, 1996; Van Os et al., 1994, 1995, 1996b; Verdoux et al., 1996).

Ethnic group. The findings give a necessarily complex picture of the outcome of psychosis in people of Caribbean origin resident in the United Kingdom, compared to white people. There was better prognosis with regard to clinical outcome in terms of symptom severity and course of illness and with regard to depression/self-harm. However, there was poorer prognosis with regard to outcomes more dependent on social factors such as imprisonment over the course of the follow-up period. This picture was confirmed when treatments received over the follow-up were compared between African-Caribbean and white patients (Table 11.4): African-Caribbean patients were more likely to have been admitted under a section of the Mental Health Act over the follow-up period, but less likely to have received antidepressants or psychotherapy.

Gender. Women had more favourable indices of course and outcome. There was no evidence for large or significant interaction with DSM-III–R diagnostic category, with the exception of "time living independently", where the effect of sex was confined to the broadly defined DSM-III–R schizophrenic category. To examine to what degree the sex–outcome differences could be explained by other variables associated both with sex and outcome, we adjusted the sex–outcome association for each potential

TABLE 11.3
Associations* Between Predictors And Outcome Dimensions

Predictor	Outcome dimension						Diagnostic interaction
	Negative symptoms/ disability	Illness severity	Time living independently	Unemployment	Imprisonment/ Vagrancy	Depression/ Self-harm	
Sex							
Men vs. women	↓	↓	↓	↓	=	=	No interaction
Ethnic group							
African-Caribbean vs. British white	=	↑	=	=	↑	↑	Stronger effect sizes in affective psychoses
Life events (LE)							
LE+ vs. LE−	=	↑	↑	=	=	=	Stronger effect sizes in affective psychoses
Family history							
Higher schizophrenia score	↓	↓	=	=	=	=	Stronger effect sizes in schizophrenia
Higher affective disorder score	=	=	=	=	=	=	
Premorbid adjustment							
Higher Philips' scale score**	↓	↓	=	↓	=	=	No interaction

(Table 11.3 continued overleaf)

143

						Stronger effect sizes in schizophrenia
Cerebral ventricle size						
Larger sylvian fissures volume	→	=	=	=	=	
Larger lateral ventricle volume	=	=	=	=	=	
Larger third ventricle volume	→	=	=	=	=	No interaction
Psychopathology						
Higher insidious–blunting score	→	→	=	#	#	
Higher delusions–hallucinations score	=	→	=	#	#	
Higher inappropriate–catatonia score	→	=	=	#		
Higher mania score	↑	↑	=	#	#	
Higher depression score	=	=	=	#	#	
Higher paranoid delusions score	=	→	=	#	#	
Higher lack of insight score	=	→	→	#	#	

* For details regarding exact effect sizes, the reader is referred to McKenzie et al., 1995; Navarro et al., 1996; Van Os et al., 1994, 1995, 1996b; Verdoux et al., 1996.

↓ Evidence for statistically significantly poorer outcome.

↑ Evidence for statistically significantly better outcome.

\# Analyses in progress.

** Higher score indicates poorer premorbid adjustment.

TABLE 11.4
Ethnic Group And Treatment Received Over The Follow-up Period

Treatment variable*	African-Caribbean group (SD or %)	British-White group (SD or %)	Difference (95% CI†)
Antidepressants ever	7/53 (13.2%)	20/60 (33.3%)	−20.1% (−35.1 to −5.1)
Lithium ever	13/53 (24.5%)	21/60 (35%)	−10.5% (−27.2 to 6.3)
Time on antipsychotics	63.8 (31.1)	59.8 (38.7)	4.0 (−9.2 to 17.2)
Involuntary admission ever‡	33/40 (82.3%)	16/37 (43.2%)	39.3% (19.4 to 59.1)
Rehabilitation ever	11/53 (20.8%)	10/59 (17.0%)	3.8% (−10.7 to 18.3)
Psychotherapy ever	1/53 (1.9%)	9/60 (15.0%)	−13.1% (−22.9 to −3.4)

*Continuous variables: mean (geometric mean for log-transformed distributions); binary variables: proportions.
†Exact confidence intervals.
‡Among those who were readmitted only.

explanatory variable separately for the four main outcome dimensions, using the measure in each outcome dimension with the strongest association with sex (Fig. 11.1; time living independently for DSM-III-R category of schizophrenia only).

Between 10% and 40% of the sex–outcome association was explained by third variables, especially marital and occupational adjustment, clinical expression of psychosis and negative symptoms, and age and type of onset. Adjustment for these six variables together reduced the sex–outcome associations as follows: non-remitting course: 33%; negative symptoms over the follow-up period: 59%; employment status at follows-up: 44%; and time living independently: 17%.

Other social and biological predictors. Although there was some variation across the different outcome dimensions, the results were relatively straightforward. Life events were associated with a less severe, good-outcome illness, whereas high familial morbid risk for schizophrenia, early developmental deviance, and enlarged cerebral ventricles predicted a more severe illness, as evidenced by a more deteriorated course.

DISCUSSION

Gender

Our results suggest that: (1) women have a more favourable illness course than men, regardless of outcome dimension; (2) although women are less likely to meet criteria for stringently defined schizophrenia, the difference in outcome is not diagnosis specific, with the exception of time living

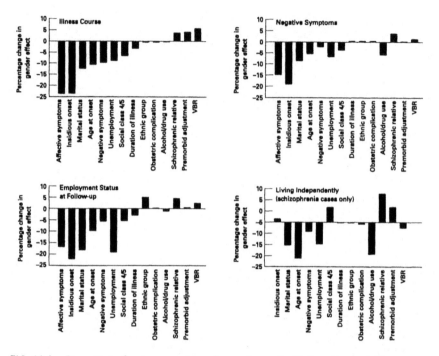

FIG. 11.1.   Percentage of outcome variance for gender explicable by other variables.

independently; (3) 20%–60% of the sex–outcome association can be explained by sex differences in social and illness characteristics.

We can now combine the findings presented in Chapters 4 and 5, with the longitudinal findings presented here. The excess of male patients found in samples of patients with "six-month" DSM-III/III–R schizophrenia will be much reduced if other, less restrictive, definitions of schizophrenia are used. As women have a better outcome (see also Angermeyer, Kuhn, & Goldstein, 1990; Bardenstein & McGlashan, 1990), the relatively unfavourable outcome in DSM-III/III–R schizophrenia as compared with the ICD construct (Brockington et al., 1978) reflects, at least in part, sex differences in the baseline presentation of schizophrenia.

The issues pertaining to sex, diagnostic variation, and outcome are summarised in Fig. 11.2. By including samples with a wide range of clinical expression of psychotic illness, the outcome variance found will be greater, and the sex distribution will be less skewed.

Our analyses showed that between 20%–60% of the sex effect on outcome could be explained by other variables. Of course, adjusting for premorbid, social, and illness characteristics does not really "explain" anything; all these characteristics presumably have their origin in one or

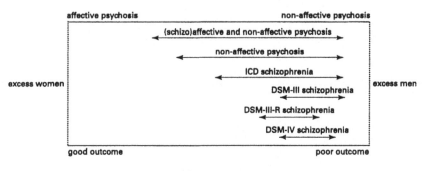

FIG. 11.2.   Relationship between diagnosis, outcome, and gender.

more latent variables. However, the fact that these variables accounted for such a large part of the sex effect does show us the direction in which to look. For example, the biological processes underlying clinical expression of illness, such as negative symptoms, may be more frequent in male patients. Similarly, attenuated neurodevelopment, resulting in poor social and occupational adjustment, may also preferentially affect men (Castle & Murray, 1991).

Ethnic group

Our study, and others before us (Harder et al., 1981; Vaillant, 1964), showed that the presence of environmental precipitants before the onset of psychosis ("life events") predict better prognosis. The better prognosis in African-Caribbeans that we have demonstrated may be due to an excess of illness with social precipitants; previous studies (Birchwood et al., 1992; Sugarman, 1992) may have failed to show the relatively good prognosis for African-Caribbeans with psychosis because of the confounding effect of social class.

However, despite favourable symptom and course indices, African-Caribbeans in south London were still more likely to be admitted under a section of the Mental Health Act, and more likely to have been in jail, but spent similar amounts of time in hospital as white patients. Our study suggests that this was not always related to the clinical state of the patient.

This is the first prospective study to show ethnic differences in self-harm in a psychotic sample. African-Caribbeans with psychosis are less at risk of self-harm than Whites, but the increasing incidence of self-harm in the wider African-Caribbean population (Raleigh & Balarajan, 1982) may result in attenuation of the protective effect conferred by ethnic group.

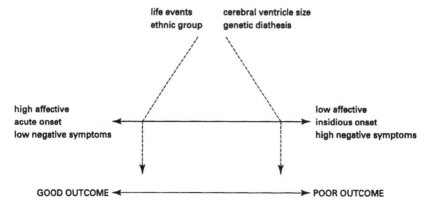

FIG. 11.3. Dimensional model of psychosis in terms of outcome.

Other social and biological predictors

In Chapter 1, we suggested that biological and social risk factors for the onset of psychosis such as life events, family history, cerebral ventricle size, and developmental deviance are not specific to any particular diagnostic category. On the basis of the findings from the Camberwell Collaborative Psychosis Study, we conclude that there is similarly little evidence that any risk factor for outcome of psychotic illness is specific to any diagnostic category within the functional psychoses. However, we have provided evidence that the magnitude of these risk factors for poor- and good-outcome illness varies as a function of baseline psychopathology, such that the life events/ethnic group association is more evident at the affective end of the spectrum, and the associations between outcome and familial morbid risk and cerebral ventricle size at the non-affective end. This is presented graphically in Fig. 11.3.

Previously, similar distinctions have been made within the diagnostic category of schizophrenia (Robins & Guze, 1970; Crow, 1980; Murray et al., 1992). We believe, however, that the current evidence favours a continuum of psychosis with several psychopathological dimensions across all diagnostic categories, including the affective disorders (see Fig. 11.3). This issue is discussed further in Chapter 12.

CHAPTER TWELVE

Summary and conclusions

We have described the epidemiology of schizophrenia, schizophrenia-like, and manic illnesses as seen in south London. Here we review the main findings, and place them in the context of the broader literature.

PATIENTS TREATED WITH OR WITHOUT ADMISSION

Over the period of 20 years from 1965 to 1984, the proportion of first-onset schizophrenics who were not admitted to hospital remained remarkably similar at around 20%. This surprised us, given the increasing emphasis on care in the community over this period. However, the combination of a stable proportion of patients being treated in the community with an increasing incidence of psychosis goes some way to explain why there has been such difficulty in running the Mental Health Services in London with a steadily reducing number of available hospital beds (Powell, Hollander, & Tobiansky, 1995).

Certain characteristics of patients predicted admission. The bizarre or behaviourally disturbed and those threatening violence to themselves or others were especially likely to be admitted. Indeed, non-specific positive symptoms such as persecutory or grandiose delusions, or any hallucination, were more likely to provoke admission than were those symptoms considered more "pathognomonic" of schizophrenia. This is consonant with the evidence that it was manic, schizoaffective, and schizophreniform

149

patients who were most likely to be admitted. These findings imply that the currently fashionable studies of schizophrenic patients during their first hospital admission are not only likely to be unrepresentative, but also likely to be unrepresentative in predictable ways.

CRIMINAL OR VIOLENT BEHAVIOUR

There has been much public concern in recent years over the number of violent acts committed by schizophrenia sufferers in the UK. Our study shows that men with schizophrenia do not have an overall increased risk of criminality compared to men with other psychiatric disorders. However, their risk of being convicted for a violent offence is at least twice that of men with non-psychotic disorders. Women with schizophrenia have an increased risk of any conviction. Acquiring a criminal record was more likely in the presence of unemployment, lower social class, substance abuse, African-Caribbean ethnicity, and also in the later years of the study; it was less likely if the individual was married, working, or female. All of these variables had stronger predictive effects for criminality, than did the presence of psychosis.

Thus, social variables remain the strongest predictors of criminal behaviour in those with mental illness but additional risk is also conveyed by psychosis itself. Schizophrenia does make a contribution to criminal behaviour, especially violent offending. The presence of schizophrenia also increased the risk of post-illness conviction by nearly twofold. Survival analysis showed that previous conviction, ethnicity, gender, and substance abuse, but not schizophrenia, remained independent predictors of post-illness conviction; the strongest predictor was a previous conviction. Thus, our findings confirm that there is an association between schizophrenia and crime but put it in its correct context: people with schizophrenia are responsible for only a very small proportion of the overall crime.

Nevertheless, the influence of African-Caribbean ethnicity on conviction rates among schizophrenic patients is of obvious concern. Not only are African-Caribbean people living in the UK at considerably greater risk of schizophrenia than those of other ethnic origins, but they have higher rates of criminal conviction than other ethnic groups in the UK. Our findings raise disturbing questions about the relationship between ethnicity, schizophrenia, and criminal conviction; no doubt excess social deprivation, and bias within the criminal justice system, partly account for our findings. However, the study also raises the possible contribution of illness-related factors, particularly in young African-Caribbeans with schizophrenia.

GENDER DIFFERENCES

Our findings of a difference in the mean age at onset between men and women with non-affective functional psychotic disorders recapitulate numerous prior reports of such differences. However, the sampling frame allowed us to move a step forward, in that patients were selected independent of diagnosis or age at onset. We were able to confirm that the later onset of schizophrenia in women is not an artifact of choice of diagnostic criteria, in that the effect was robust to stringency of diagnosis.

In defining the main contributions to age at onset, we found robust independent associations between early onset and single marital status, as well as poor premorbid work adjustment; these factors operated in much the same way for both men and women. Sex itself was found to be an independent predictor of early illness onset, even after controlling for other premorbid variables.

That both married men and women had a later mean onset of illness is hardly surprising, and probably reflects a combination of better premorbid functioning in individuals with a later onset; a longer illness-free period in which to marry; and possibly some "protective" effect of marriage itself. When only single individuals were considered, the sex difference in onset was enhanced. This is again in line with the notion that there is a severe early-onset form of illness associated with premorbid and psychosocial impairment, to which males are particularly prone.

The age-at-onset distribution curves for men and women with non-affective psychotic disorders are not isomorphic. Thus, it is not as though the curve for women is merely shifted to the right, as would be predicted by a simple explanation for the difference in onset in terms of some factor delaying onset in women. The different distributions demand a more sophisticated explanatory hypothesis. One possibility is that there are different forms of illness with different mean ages of onset, and to which males and females are differentially prone. For example, we found that males were more prone to the neurodevelopmental form of illness. Women were not free of risk for such an illness, merely that they were less likely to get it. In support of this conclusion, we found that, in terms of premorbid adjustment, it was males with an early onset of illness who fared worst, although early-onset females were also more impaired than their late-onset counterparts.

A second difference between men and women lay in the proportion who met various criteria for schizophrenia. Thus, while the incidence of schizophrenia appeared relatively equal in men and women when broad criteria for schizophrenia were used, DSM-III criteria preferentially excluded women; this arose partly because of the age cut-off in DSM-III and partly because of its requirement of six months of continuing illness.

As a consequence, narrowly defined schizophrenia appeared at least twice as common in males as in females.

TRENDS IN INCIDENCE

After apparently remaining relatively constant over the first half of this century, reports began to appear in the 1980s suggesting a decline in the incidence of schizophrenia in a number of developed countries (Der et al., 1990). Although this may have been in part due to changes in the diagnostic concept or in patterns of care (Kendell et al., 1993), birth cohort studies in the UK suggest that it is in part a genuine decline (Takei, Lewis, Sham, & Murray, 1996).

Consequently, we had expected to see a decline in the incidence of schizophrenia in Camberwell parallel to the decline in both national first admissions and regional first contacts of patients with schizophrenia. However, we found an increase in the incidence of first contact schizophrenia in Camberwell over the 20 year period, 1965–1984. This was not accounted for by any shift in diagnostic habits towards rediagnosing as schizophrenic patients who would previously have been regarded as suffering from mania. Indeed, the incidence of mania also increased over this period.

ETHNICITY

The primary reason for the increase in the incidence of both schizophrenia and mania over the 20-year period was the influx into Camberwell of migrants from the Caribbean. Thus, our study confirms reports that African-Caribbean people in the UK have a high incidence not only of schizophrenia but also of mania. The fact that the incidence of both these disorders is raised in this population suggests that there exist risk-increasing factors that are common to both conditions. Certainly, the causes of the epidemic of psychosis in African-Caribbeans (and indeed Africans, as we have shown in Chapter 10) living in the UK merits urgent investigation.

Two recent findings may be of relevance. First, Hutchison and colleagues (1996) have confirmed the previous evidence of Sugarman and Crawford (1993) that the siblings (but not the parents) of second generation African-Caribbean psychotic patients have a much higher risk of psychosis than the siblings of white psychotic patients; this implies the operation of an environmental factor possibly exerting its effect, especially upon vulnerable families. A second but compatible finding comes from G. Kirov and R. M. Murray (personal communication, June, 1996) who have shown that in south London, African and African-Caribbean patients who are receiving lithium are more likely than their white counterparts to show predominantly manic episodes and mood-incongruent delusions and less likely to show suicidal ideas or actions. Similarly, a recent American study has found that African-Americans with psychosis are more likely than Whites to show Schneiderian first-rank symptoms and consequently to receive a diagnosis of schizophrenia; these authors therefore raise the question of whether schizophrenia is overdiagnosed in the black population and affective psychotic disorders underdiagnosed.

An integration of these two pieces of evidence might suggest that environmental pressures associated with the disadvantageous social position of the African-Caribbean population within British society results in psychotic breakdown among those at particular familial risk of disorder; the resultant psychosis often presents an affective, mainly manic picture, but may also show Schneiderian or mood-incongruent features and result in the affected individual receiving a diagnosis of schizophrenia. This hypothesis is also compatible with the evidence presented in Chapter 11 that African-Caribbean psychotic patients in south London are especially likely to show an illness course characterised by relapses and recovery.

LATE-ONSET SCHIZOPHRENIA

The relatively large differential in age of onset in the current sample reflects our inclusion of patients with a very late onset of illness; such patients have been excluded from most previous studies. Our findings reinforce the previous reports of the existence of a significant minority of patients with a late and very late onset of a schizophrenia-like illness, and show that a relatively high proportion of such patients fulfil stringent diagnostic criteria for schizophrenia. Nevertheless, we were able to delineate differences between such cases and their early-onset counterparts in terms of premorbid functioning and phenomenology; in particular thought disorder was mainly confined to the early-onset patients. Other research, as in the current study, also suggests that late-onset schizophrenia is less likely to be associated with obstetric complications (Verdoux et al., 1997) or with a high morbid risk of schizophrenia in relatives (Howard et al., 1997); in our parlance, late-onset schizophrenia appears less associated with neurodevelopmental risk factors.

How can we explain the occurrence of onset of schizophrenia relatively late in life, particularly since neurodevelopmental risk factors are rarely found in such cases? There appear to be two main possibilities. Either there exists (a) heterogeneity with neurodevelopmental abnormality having no bearing on late-onset schizophrenia, this being caused by quite different factors; or (b) dimensional differences with abnormal neurodevelopment having only a limited effect allowing the individual to remain non-psychotic until its effects are compounded by other later risk factors, or brain degeneration.

CLASSIFICATION OF PSYCHOSIS

In an ideal world, psychiatric diagnostic categories would be derived from knowledge of their distinct underlying causes, and distinct subdivisions would reflect their separate aetiologies. Unfortunately, our knowledge of psychotic conditions has not yet advanced to this point. In the absence of an aetiologically validated classification, it has been argued that predictive validity, the demonstration of a qualitative difference in outcome between two disorders, is the next most important form of validity; indeed, a high predictive validity concerning course and treatment response is good justification for a classificatory system.

Unfortunately, the so-called Kraepelinian division of the functional psychoses into schizophrenia and manic-depressive psychosis has neither aetiological nor predictive validity. It is clearly unwise to base one's entire research strategy on a categorical approach if the diagnostic boundaries remain arbitrary and subject to frequent changes. For example, even within the DSM diagnostic system, there have been repeated changes in the criteria for schizophrenia; each change includes or excludes different patients. Thus, we found that many more of the psychotic patients who presented to psychiatric services in Camberwell between 1965 and 1984 met DSM-III–R than DSM-III criteria for schizophrenia. Such boundary changes are likely to affect the comparability of research results from one DSM generation to another in a so far unquantified way. It was for such reasons that McGlashan (1988) argued that "until significant progress is made in reducing the heterogeneity of schizophrenia, its criteria should err in the direction of inclusiveness."

We therefore adopted an inclusive approach in this book. Not only did we examine the effect of using different definitions of schizophrenia, but we also included other non-affective psychoses and indeed manic disorders in many of our analyses. The wisdom of these decisions has been emphasised by our findings; for example, that mania and schizophrenia appear to be subject to some of the same risk factors. By moving away from diagnostic constructs towards a continuum of psychosis, we avoided several other methodological pitfalls. For example, the use of alternative diagnostic criteria considerably changes important demographic characteristics of our sample of "schizophrenics". Thus, as we have seen, the huge excess of male patients found meeting the "six-month long" criteria for DSM-III schizophrenia was much reduced when less restrictive definitions of schizophrenia were used.

Another advantage of the broad approach that we have used is that within-sample clinical heterogeneity, in terms of either symptom dimensions or diagnostic categories, can be examined more easily than by starting out with narrowly defined cases of schizophrenia at the extreme end of the psychosis continuum. Had we carried out the latent class analysis described in Chapter 5 on a narrowly defined sample of nuclear schizophrenics, then it is unlikely that we would have identified the three subtypes; neurodevelopmental, paranoid, and schizoaffective. The most robust of these was the "neurodevelopmental", a severe early-onset illness associated with premorbid dysfunction, negative symptomatology, a family history of schizophrenia, and obstetric complications. A paranoid subtype, with prominent paranoid ideas but less premorbid dysfunction and lower family loading for schizophrenia, was also delineated, in line with a number of other typological investigations of schizophrenia; a novel finding in the current study was an association of this subtype with winter birth, suggesting that some seasonal environmental aetiological factor (possibly a virus) might be operating in some such individuals. Finally, the finding of a group of females with prominent affective symptomatology and a family history of psychiatric illness other than schizophrenia (mostly affective disorder), lends support to the notion that some females usually labelled "schizophrenic" have an illness with links to affective disorder.

Thus, our investigation indicates that there is heterogeneity even within the concept of schizophrenia. At first sight, this might suggest that schizophrenia should be further divided into subtypes rather than as part of a continuum of psychosis. However, we do not consider that the existence of these three subtypes contradicts the view outlined earlier that psychosis should be seen as a continuum. On the contrary, as we have argued in Chapter 5, we regard these idealised subtypes as the expression within the arbitrary category of schizophrenia of dimensions which operate to a greater or lesser extent across psychosis.

The data from the Camberwell Collaborative Psychosis Study, some of which are presented in Chapter 11, lend support to this view. Thus, a family loading for schizophrenia was associated with negative symptoms, while a family loading for affective disorder was associated with a syndrome of "inappropriate–catatonia" within the schizophrenia category. Not surprisingly, a family loading for mania was associated with manic-depression (Van Os et al., 1997b). Furthermore, a familial loading for schizophrenia was associated with a lower likelihood of recovery at four-year follow-up; the effect of familial loading on outcome was greater in the schizophrenic than in the non-schizophrenic psychoses, as would be predicted by a dimensional model.

The dimensional model also gains support from the findings that adverse life events were found to be most common prior to affective psychosis although they also occurred in excess in schizophrenia. At the four-year follow-up, patients who had suffered such adversity were nearly ten times more likely to have a symptom severity of "mild" or "recovered" over most of the follow-up period. Thus, psychotic patients whose illness is reactive to life events present more frequently with affective rather than schizophrenic symptoms; such patients tend to experience frequent relapses followed by rapid recovery, even when schizophreniform in nature. Indeed, one possible explanation for the high incidence of both major psychoses that we found in African-Caribbeans in Camberwell is that they suffered an excess of psychotic illnesses consequent largely upon social adversity.

Structural brain abnormalities, as visualised on CT scan, were most common in schizophrenia but nevertheless they were also noted in those diagnosed as having affective psychoses (Jones et al., 1994b). Cerebral ventricle size was a risk factor for negative symptoms and unemployment over the follow-up period, and attenuated cognitive functioning at follow-up as assessed by the Trails test. These effects were stronger in (but not specific to) DSM-III–R schizophrenia (see Chapter 11).

Thus, the evidence from both the epidemiological studies reported in this book and that from the Camberwell Collaborative Psychosis Study, suggests that a dimensional model of psychosis fits the available data better than one based on the traditional Kraepelinian subtypes. Rather than qualitative differences, there appears to be a "dose-response" relationship between the acuteness of onset and the degree of affective symptomatology, and both risk factors and outcome. In other words, what appears to have been established is a psychopathological continuum, not discrete entities.

What appears most "valid" (at least for the time being) is a psychopathological continuum of symptom dimensions, especially dimensions of affective/non-affective, insidious/acute onset and low/high negative symptomatology. The findings suggest discrete effects working preferentially, though not exclusively, at particular ends of the continuum; that is, there is a gradient, both in terms of severity/prognosis and the magnitude of the effect of risk factors, along the continuum, rather than qualitative distinctions between categories.

References

Addonizio, G.C. (1995). Late paraphrenia. *Psychiatric Clinics of North America, 18,* 335–343.

Akiskal, H.S., Maser, J. D., Zeller, P.J., Endicot, J., Coryell, W., Keller, M., Warshaw, M., Clayton, P., & Goodwin, F. (1995). Switching from 'unipolar' to bipolar II. *Archives of General Psychiatry, 52,* 114–123.

Almeida, O.P., Howard, R., Forstl, H., & Levy, R. (1992). Should the diagnosis of late paraphrenia be abandoned? *Psychological Medicine, 22,* 11–14.

American Psychiatric Association. (1980). *Diagnostic and statistical manual for the classification of psychiatric diseases* (3rd edn). Washington DC: APA.

American Psychiatric Association. (1987). *Diagnostic and statistical manual for the classification of psychiatric diseases* (3rd edn, revised). Washington DC: APA.

American Psychiatric Association. (1994). *Diagnostic and statistical manual of mental disorders* (4th edn) (DSM-IV). Washington DC: APA.

Ames, F.R. (1991). Sex and the brain. *South African Medical Journal, 80,* 150–152.

Andreasen, N.C., Swayze, V.W., Flaum, M., Alliger, R., & Cohen, M. (1990). Ventricular abnormalities in affective disorder: Clinical and demographic correlates. *Archives of General Psychiatry, 47,* 893–900.

Angermeyer, M.C., Goldstein, J.M., & Kuhn, L. (1988). Gender differences in age at onset of schizophrenia: An overview. *European Archives of Psychiatry and Neurological Sciences, 237,* 351–364.

Angermeyer, M.C., Kuhn, L., & Goldstein, J.M. (1990). Sex and the course of schizophrenia: Differences in treated outcomes. *Schizophrenia Bulletin, 16,* 293–307.

Aylward, E., Walker, E., & Bettes, B. (1984). Intelligence in schizophrenia: A meta-analysis. *Schizophrenia Bulletin, 10,* 430–459.

Balarajan, R., Raleigh, V.S., & Botting, B. (1989). Mortality from congenital malformations in England and Wales: Variations by mother's country of birth. *Archives of Diseases in Childhood, 64,* 1457–1462.

Balarajan, R., Yuen, P., & Machin, D. (1992). Deprivation and general practitioner workload. *British Medical Journal, 304,* 116–130.

Bamrah, J.S., Freeman, H.L., & Goldberg, D.P. (1991). Epidemiology of schizophrenia in Salford, 1974–84. *British Journal of Psychiatry, 159,* 802–810.

Bardenstein, K., & McGlashan, T. (1990). Sex differences in affective, schizoaffective, and schizophrenic disorders: A review. *Schizophrenia Research, 3,* 159–72.

Barker, D.J.P. (1989). Rise and fall of Western diseases. *Nature, 338,* 371–372.

Baron, M., Gruen, R. Asnis, L., & Kane, J. (1982). Schizo-affective illness, schizophrenia and affective disorders: Morbid risk and genetic transmission. *Acta Psychiatrica Scandinavica, 65,* 253–262.

Baron, M., Gruen, R., Kane, J., & Asnis, L. (1985). Modern research criteria and the genetics of schizophrenia. *American Journal of Psychiatry, 142,* 697–701.

Bebbington, P., Hurry, J., & Tennant, C. (1981). Psychiatric disorders in selected immigrant groups in Camberwell. *Social Psychiatry, 16,* 43–51.

Bebbington, P., Brugha, T., MacCarthy, J., Potter, J., Sturt, E., Wykes, T., Katz, R., & McGuffin, P. (1988). The Camberwell Collaborative Depression Study I. Depressed probands: Adversity and the form of depression. *British Journal of Psychiatry, 152,* 754–765.

Bebbington, P., & Kuipers, L. (1988). Social influences on schizophrenia. In P. McGuffin & P. Bebbington (Eds.), *Schizophrenia: The major issue.* Heinemann: Oxford.

Bebbington, P., Wilkins, S., Jones, P.B., Foerster, A., Murray, R., Toone, B., & Lewis, S. (1993). Life events and psychosis. Initial results from the Camberwell Collaborative Psychosis Study. *British Journal of Psychiatry, 162,* 72–79.

Beiser, M., & Iacono, W. (1990). An update on the epidemiology of schizophrenia. *Canadian Journal of Psychiatry, 35,* 657–668.

Bernadt, M., & Murray, R. (1986). Psychiatric disorder, drinking and alcoholism. *British Journal of Psychiatry, 148,* 393–400.

Bertelsen, A., Harvald, B., & Hauge, M. (1977). A Danish twin study of manic depressive disorders. *British Journal of Psychiatry, 130,* 330–51.

Birchwood, M., Cochrane, R., MacMillan, F., Copestake, S., Kucharska, J., & Carris, M. (1992). The influence of ethnicity and family structure on relapse in first-episode schizophrenia. *British Journal of Psychiatry, 161,* 783–790.

Bland, R.C. (1977). Demographic aspects of functional psychoses in Canada. *Acta Psychiatrica Scandinavica, 55,* 369–380.

Bleuler, E. (1943). Die spatschizophrenen Krankheitsbilder (The clinical picture in late schizophrenia). *Fortschr. Neurol. Psychiat., 15,* 259–290.

Bradbury, T.N., & Miller, G.A. (1985). Season of birth in schizophrenia: A review of evidence, methodology, and aetiology. *Psychological Bulletin, 98,* 569–594.

Breier, A., Schreiber, J.L., & Dyer, J. (1992). Course of illness and predictors of outcome in chronic schizophrenia: Implications for pathophysiology. *British Journal of Psychiatry 161,* (Suppl. 18), 38–42.

Breslow N.E., & Day N.E. (1987). *Statistical methods in cancer research,* vol 1. Lyon: WHO.

Brockington, I., Kendell, R.E., & Leff, J. (1978). Definitions of schizophrenia: Concordance and prediction of outcome. *Psychological Medicine, 8,* 387–398.

Brockington, I., Kendell, R., & Wainwright, S. (1980a). Depressed patients with schizophrenic or paranoid symptoms. *Psychological Medicine, 10,* 665–675.

Brockington, I., Wainwright, S., & Kendell, R. (1980b). Manic patients with schizophrenic or paranoid symptoms. *Psychological Medicine, 10,* 73–83.

Brockington, I., Roper, A., Edmunds, E., Kaufman, C., & Meltzer, H. (1992). A longitudinal psychopathological schedule. *Psychological Medicine, 22,* 1035–43.

Brodaty, H., Harris, L., Peters, K., Wilhelm, K., Hickie, I., Boyce, P., Mitchell, P., Parker, G., & Eyer, S.K. (1993). Prognosis of depression in the elderly. *British Journal of Psychiatry, 163*, 589–596.

Brown, C. (1984). *Black and white Britain: The third PSI survey*. London: Heinemann.

Brown, G.W., & Harris, T.O. (1978). *Social origins of depression*. London: Tavistock.

Burke, A. (1989). Psychiatric practice and ethnic minorities. In J.K. Cruickshank & D.G. Beevers (Eds.), *Ethnic factors in health and disease*. London: Wright.

Castle, D.J., & Murray, R.M. (1991). The neurodevelopmental basis of sex differences in schizophrenia. *Psychological Medicine, 21*, 565–575.

Castle, D., Wessely, S., Der, G. & Murray, R. (1991). The incidence of operationally defined schizophrenia in Camberwell, 1965 to 1984. *British Journal of Psychiatry, 159*, 790–794.

Castle, D.J., & Howard, R. (1992). What do we know about the aetiology of late-onset schizophrenia? *European Psychiatry, 7*, 99–108.

Castle, D.J., & Murray, R.M. (1993). The epidemiology of late-onset schizophrenia. *Schizophrenia Bulletin, 19*, 691–700.

Castle, D., Scott, K., Wessely, S., & Murray, R. (1993). Does social deprivation during gestation and early life predispose to later schizophrenia? *Social Psychiatry and Psychiatric Epidemiology, 28*, 1–4.

Castle, D.J., Sham, P., Wessely, S., & Murray, R.M. (1994). The subtyping of schizophrenia in men and women: A latent class analysis. *Psychological Medicine, 24*, 41–51.

Castle, D.J., Abel, K., Takei, N., & Murray, R.M. (1995). Gender differences in schizophrenia: Hormonal effects, or subtypes? *Schizophrenia Bulletin, 21*, 1–12.

Castle, D.J., & Ames, F.R. (1996) Cannabis and the brain. *Australian and New Zealand Journal of Psychiatry, 30*, 179–183.

Castle, D.J., Wessely, S., Howard, R., & Murray, R.M. (1997). Schizophrenia with onset at the extremes of adult life. *International Journal of Geriatric Psychiatry, 12*, 712–717.

Christenson, R., & Blazer, D. (1984). Epidemiology of persecutory ideation in an elderly population in the community. *American Journal of Psychiatry, 141*, 59–67.

Clogg, C.C. (1977). *Unrestricted and restricted maximum likelihood latent structure analysis: A manual for users*. University Park, PA: Population Issues Research Office.

Clogg, C.C., & Goodman, L.A. (1985). Simultaneous latent structure analysis in several groups. In N.B. Tuma. (Ed.), *Sociological methodology*. San Francisco: Jossey-Bass.

Cochrane, R., & Bal, R. (1989). Mental hospital admission rates of immigrants to England: A comparison of 1971 and 1981. *Social Psychiatry, 24*, 2–11.

Coid, J. (1983). The epidemiology of abnormal homicide and homicide followed by suicide. *Psychological Medicine, 13*, 855–860.

Commission for Racial Equality. (1992). *Cautions v. prosecutions: Ethnic monitoring of juveniles by seven police forces*. London: Commission for Racial Equality.

Cooper, J.E., Kendell, R.E., Gurland, B.J., Sharpe, L., Copeland J.R.M., & Simon, R. (1972). *Psychiatric diagnosis in New York and London. Maudsley Monograph no. 20.* London: Oxford University Press.

Cooper, J., Goodhead, D., Craig, T., Harris, M., Howards, J., & Korer, J. (1987). The incidence of schizophrenia in Nottingham. *British Journal of Psychiatry, 151*, 619–26.

Coryell, W., & Zimmerman, M. (1988). The heritability of schizophrenia and schizoaffective disorder. *Archives of General Psychiatry, 45*, 323–327.

Coryell, W., Endicott, J., & Keller, M. (1990a). Outcome of patients with chronic affective disorder: A five year follow-up. *American Journal of Psychiatry, 147*, 1627–1633.

Coryell, W., Keller, M., Lavori, P., & Endicott, J. (1990b). Affective syndromes, psychotic features, and prognosis. I: Depression. *Archives of General Psychiatry, 47*, 651–657.

Coryell, W., Keller, M., Lavori, P., & Endicott, J. (1990c). Affective syndromes, psychotic features, and prognosis. II: Mania. *Archives of General Psychiatry, 47*, 658–662.

Cowell, P.E., Kostianovsky, D.J., Gur, R.C., Turetsky, B.I., & Gur, R.E. (1996). Sex differences in neuranatomical and clinical correlations in schizophrenia. *American Journal of Psychiatry, 153,* 799–805.

Crow, T.J. (1980). Molecular pathology of schizophrenia: More than one disease. *British Medical Journal, 280,* 66–68.

Crow, T.J. (1985). The two-syndrome concept: Origin and current status. *Schizophrenia Bulletin, 11,* 471–85.

Crow, I. (1987). Black people and criminal justice in the U.K. *Howard Journal of Criminal Justice, 26,* 303–314.

Crow, T.J. (1990). Trends in schizophrenia. *Lancet, 335,* 851.

Cruickshank, J., & Beevers, D. (1989). Migration, ethnicity, health and disease. In J. Cruickshank & D. Beevers (Eds.), *Ethnic factors in health and disease.* London: Wright.

De Alarçon, J., Seagroatt, V., & Goldacre, M. (1990). Trends in schizophrenia. *Lancet, 335,* 852–53.

Dean, G., Walsh, D., Downing, H., & Shelley, E. (1981). First admissions of native-born and immigrants to psychiatric hospitals in South-East England 1976. *British Journal of Psychiatry, 139,* 506–512.

Dean, C., & Gadd, E.M. (1990). Home treatment for acute psychiatric illness. *British Medical Journal, 301,* 1021–1023.

Deister, A., & Marneros, A. (1993). Predicting the long-term outcome of affective disorders. *Acta Psychiatrica Scandinavica, 88,* 174–177.

Der, G., & Bebbington, P. (1987). Depression in inner London: A register study. *Social Psychiatry, 22,* 73–84.

Der, G., Gupta, S., & Murray R. (1990). Is schizophrenia disappearing? *Lancet, 335,* 513–516.

Dickson, W.E., & Kendell, R.E. (1986). Does maintenance lithium therapy prevent ordinary clinical conditions? *Psychological Medicine, 16,* 521–530.

Dohrenwend, B.P., Shrout, P.E., Link, B.G., Skodol, A.E., & Stueve, A. (1995). Life events and other possible psychosocial risk factors for episodes of schizophrenia and major depression: A case–control study. In C. M. Mazure (Ed.), *Does stress cause psychiatric illness?* Washington, DC: American Psychiatric Press.

Done, J., Sacker, A., & Crow, T.J. (1994). Childhood antecedents of schizophrenia and affective illness: Intellectual performance at ages 7 and 11. *Schizophrenia Research, 11,* 96–97.

Duggan, C., Lee, A.S., & Murray R.M. (1990). Does personality predict long-term outcome in depression? *British Journal of Psychiatry, 1990, 157,* 19–25.

Eagles, J., & Whalley, L. (1985). Decline in the diagnosis of schizophrenia among first admissions to Scottish mental hospitals from 1969–1978. *British Journal of Psychiatry, 146,* 151–154.

Eagles, J.M., Hunter, D., & McCance, C. (1988). Decline in the diagnosis of schizophrenia among first contacts with psychiatric services in North East Scotland, 1969–1984. *British Journal of Psychiatry, 152,* 793–798.

Eagles, J.M. (1991). The relationship between schizophrenia and immigration. Are there alternative hypotheses? *British Journal of Psychiatry, 159,* 783–789.

Eagles, J.M. (1993). Incidence and epidemiology of schizophrenia in Denmark. *British Journal of Psychiatry, 162,* 268–269.

Eaton, W.W. (1980). A formal theory of selection for schizophrenia. *American Journal of Sociology, 86,* 149–158.

Eaton, W. (1985). Epidemiology of schizophrenia. *Epidemiologic Reviews, 7,* 105–126.

Eaton, W.W., Mortensen, P.B., Herrman, H., Freeman, H., Bilker, W., Burgess, P., & Wooff, K. (1992). Long-term course of hospitalisation for schizophrenia: Part 1. Risk for rehospitalisation. *Schizophrenia Bulletin, 18,* 217–228

Elkis, H., Friedman, L., Wise, A., & Meltzer, H. (1995). Meta-analyses of studies of ventricular enlargement and cortical sulcal prominence in mood disorders. *Archives of General Psychiatry, 52*, 735–746.

Farmer, A.E., McGuffin, P., & Spitznagel, E.L. (1983). Heterogeneity in schizophrenia: A cluster-analytic approach. *Psychiatry Research, 8*, 1–12.

Farmer, A., Wessely, S., Castle, D., & McGuffin, P. (1992). Methodological issues in using a polydiagnostic approach to define psychotic illness. *British Journal of Psychiatry, 161*, 824–830.

Faroane, S.V., Chen, W.J., Goldstein, J.M., & Tsuang, M.T. (1994). Gender differences in age at onset of schizophrenia. *British Journal of Psychiatry, 164*, 625–629.

Farrington, D. (1973). Self-reports of deviant behaviour: predictive and stable? *Journal of Criminal Law and Criminology, 64*, 99–110.

Farrington, D. (1981). The prevalence of convictions. *British Journal of Criminology, 21*, 173–175.

Farrington, D. (1988). Studying changes within individuals: The causes of offending. In M. Rutter (Ed.), *Studies of psychosocial risk: The power of longitudinal data.* Cambridge: Cambridge University Press.

Farrington, D. (1990). Age, period, cohort and offending. In D. Gottfriedson & R. Clarke (Eds.), *Policy and theory in criminal justice.* Cambridge Studies in Criminology No. 52. Aldershot: Avebury.

Farrington, D. & West, D. (1990). The Cambridge study in delinquent development: A long-term follow-up of 411 London males. In H. Kerner & G. Kaiser (Eds.), *Kriminalität: Persönlichkeit, Lebensgeschichte und Verhalten.* Berlin: Springer Verlag.

Farrington, D. (1993). The psychological milieu of the offender. In J. Gunn & P. Taylor (Eds.), *Forensic Psychiatry: Clinical, ethical and legal issues.* London: Heinemann.

Feighner, J.P., Robins, E, Guze, S.B., Woodruff, R., Winokur, G., & Munoz, R. (1972). Diagnostic criteria for use in psychiatric research. *Archives of General Psychiatry, 26*, 57–63.

Folnegovic, Z., Folnegovic-Šmalc, V., & Kulcar, Z. (1990). The incidence of schizophrenia in Croatia. *British Journal of Psychiatry, 156*, 363–365.

Freeman, H. (1994) Schizophrenia and city residence. *British Journal of Psychiatry, 164* (suppl. 23), 39–50.

Gardner, M., & Altman, D. (1989). *Statistics with confidence.* London: British Medical Journal.

Geddes, J.R., Black, R.J., Whalley, L.J., & Eagles, J.M. (1993). Persistence of the decline of the diagnosis of schizophrenia among first admissions to Scottish hospitals from 1969 to 1988. *British Journal of Psychiatry, 163*, 620–626.

Geddes, J.R., & Lawrie, S.M. (1995). Obstetric complications and schizophrenia: A meta-analysis. *British Journal of Psychiatry, 167*, 786–793.

Gershon, E., Mark, A., Cohen, N., Belizon, N. Baron, M., & Knobe, K.E. (1975). Transmitted factors in the morbid risk of affective disorders: A controlled study. *Journal of Psychiatry Research, 12*, 283–299.

Gershon, E.S., DeLisi, L.E., Hamovit, J., Nurnberger, J.I., Maxwell, M.E., Schreiber, J., Dauphinais, D., Dingman, C.W., & Guroff, J.J. (1988). A controlled family study of chronic psychoses: Schizophrenia and schizo-affective disorder. *Archives of General Psychiatry, 45*, 328–336.

Giovannoni, J., & Gurel, L. (1967). Socially disruptive behaviour of ex-mental patients. *Archives of General Psychiatry 17*, 146–153.

Glover, G. (1989a). The pattern of psychiatric admissions of Caribbean-born immigrants in London. *Social Psychiatry, 24*, 49–56.

Glover, G. (1989b). Why is there a high rate of schizophrenia in British Afro-Caribbeans? *British Journal Hospital Medicine, 42,* 48–51.

Goldacre, M., Shiwatch, R., & Yeates, D. (1994). Estimating incidence and prevalence of treated psychiatric disorders from routine statistics: The example of schizophrenia in Oxfordshire. *Journal of Epidemiology and Community Health, 48,* 318–322.

Goldberg, D., & Huxley, P. (1980). *Mental illness in the community.* London: Tavistock.

Goldstein, J.M., Santangelo, S.L., Simpson, J.C., & Tsuang, M.T. (1990). The role of gender in identifying subtypes of schizophrenia: A latent class approach. *Schizophrenia Bulletin, 16,* 263–275.

Gottesman, I.I., & Shields, J. (1982). *Schizophrenia: The epigenetic puzzle.* Cambridge: Cambridge University Press

Graham, P.M. (1990). Trends in schizophrenia. *Lancet, 335,* 852.

Green, B.F. (1951). A general solution of the latent class model of latent structure analysis and latent profile analysis. *Psychometrika, 16,* 151–166.

Hafner, H., & Gattaz, W.F. (1991). Is schizophrenia disappearing? *European Archives of Psychiatry and Clinical Neuroscience, 240,* 374–376.

Hafner, H., Behrens, S., De Vry, J., & Gattaz, W.F. (1991). An animal model for the effects of estradiol on dopamine-mediated behaviour: Implications for sex differences in schizophrenia. *Psychiatry Research, 38,* 125–134.

Hambrecht, M., Maurer, K., Hafner, H., & Sartorius, N. (1992). Transnational stability of gender differences in schizophrenia. *European Archives of Psychiatry and Neurological Sciences, 242,* 6–12.

Hamilton, M. (1960). A rating scale for depression. *Journal of Neurology, Neurosurgery and Psychiatry, 23,* 56–58.

Harder, D., Gift, T.E., Strauss, J.S., Ritzler, B.A., & Kokes, R.F. (1981). Life events and two-year outcome in schizophrenia. *Journal of Consulting and Clinical Psychology, 49,* 619–626.

Harder, D., Greenwald, D., Ritzler, B., Strauss, J., Kokes, R., & Gift, T. (1990). Prediction of outcome among adult psychiatric first-admissions. *Journal of Clinical Psychology, 46,* 119–129.

Harris, M.J., & Jeste, M.J. (1988). Late onset schizophrenia: An overview. *Schizophrenia Bulletin, 14,* 39–55.

Harrison, G., Owens, D., Holton, A., Neilson, D., & Boot, D. (1988). A prospective study of severe mental disorder in Afro-Caribbean patients. *Psychological Medicine, 18,* 643–657.

Harrison, G. (1989). A perspective from Nottingham, UK. In J. Cruickshank & D. Beevers (Eds.), *Ethnic factors in health and disease.* London: Wright.

Harrison, G., Holten, A., Nielson, D., Owens, D., & Boot, D. (1989). Severe mental disorders in Afro-Caribbean patients: Some social, demographic, and service factors. *Psychological Medicine, 19,* 683–696.

Harrison, G. (1990). Searching for the causes of schizophrenia: The role of migrant studies. *Schizophrenia Bulletin, 16,* 663–671.

Harrison, G., Cooper, J., & Gancarczyk, R. (1991). Changes in the administrative incidence of schizophrenia. *British Journal of Psychiatry, 159,* 811–816.

Harvey, I., Williams, M., McGuffin, P., & Toone, B. (1990). The functional psychoses in Afro-Caribbeans. *British Journal of Psychiatry, 157,* 515–522.

Harvey, I., Persaud, R., Ron, M.A., Barker, G., & Murray, R.M. (1994). Volumetric MRI measures in bipolars compared with schizophrenics and healthy controls. *Psychological Medicine, 4,* 689–699.

Herbert, M.E., & Jacobsen, S. (1967). Late paraphrenia. *British Journal of Psychiatry, 113,* 461–469.

Hickling, F., & Rodgers–Johnson, P. (1995). The incidence of first contact schizophrenia in Jamaica. *British Journal of Psychiatry, 167,* 193–196.

Hindelang, M. (1983). Race and involvement in crime. *American Sociological Review, 43,* 93–109.

Hodgins, S. (1992). Mental disorder, intellectual deficiency, and crime: Evidence from a birth cohort. *Archives of General Psychiatry, 49,* 476–483.

Hodgins, S., Mednick, S., Brennan, P., Schulsinger, F., & Engberg, M. (1996). Mental disorder and crime: Evidence from a Danish birth cohort. *Archives of General Psychiatry, 53,* 489–496.

Home Office Statistical Bulletin. (1989). *Crime statistics for the Metropolitan Police District by ethnic group. 1987: Victims, suspects and those arrested.* London: Home Office Statistical Department.

Howard, R.M., Castle, D., O'Brien, J., Almeida, O., & Levy, R. (1992). Permeable walls, floors, ceilings and doors: Partition delusions in late paraphrenia. *International Journal of Geriatric Psychiatry, 7,* 719–724.

Howard, R.M., Castle, D., Wessely, S., & Murray, R.M. (1993). A comparison study of 470 cases of early-onset and late-onset schizophrenia. *British Journal of Psychiatry, 163,* 352–357.

Howard, R., Graham, C., Sham, P., Dennehy, J., Castle, D., Levy, R., & Murray, R. (1997). A controlled family study of late-onset non-affective psychosis (late paraphrenia). *British Journal of Psychiatry, 170,* 511–514.

Huizinga, D., & Elliot, D. (1986). Reassessing the reliability and validity of self-report measures. *Journal of Quantitative Criminology, 2,* 293–327.

Humphreys, M., Johnstone, E., MacMillan, J., & Taylor, P. (1992). Dangerous behaviour preceding first admissions for schizophrenia. *British Journal of Psychiatry, 161,* 501–505.

Hutchinson, G., Takei, N., Fahy, T., Bhugra, D., Moran, P., McKenzie, K., & Leff, J. (1996). Morbid risk for schizophrenia in African–Caribbean and white psychotic patients. *British Journal of Psychiatry, 169,* 776–780.

Iager, A.C., Kirch, D.G., & Wyatt, R.J. (1985). A negative symptom rating scale. *Psychiatry Research, 16,* 27–36.

Inghe, G. (1941). Mental abnormalities among criminals. *Acta Psychiatrica Neurologica Scandinavica, 16,* 421–458.

Institute of Psychiatry Training Committee (1973). *Notes on eliciting and recording clinical information.* Oxford: Oxford University Press.

Jablensky, A., Schwartz, R., & Tomov, T. (1980). WHO collaborative study of impairments and disabilities associated with schizophrenic disorders. A preliminary communication. Objective and methods. *Acta Psychiatrica Scandinavica, suppl. 285,* 152–163.

Jablensky, A., Sartorius, N., & Ernberg, G. (1992). Schizophrenia: Manifestations, incidence and course in different cultures. *Psychological Medicine,* monograph supplement 20. Cambridge: Cambridge University Press.

Jablensky, A. (1993). The epidemiology of schizophrenia. *Current Opinion in Psychiatry, 6,* 43–52.

Jablensky, A., & Cole, S.W. (1997). Is the earlier age at onset of schizophrenia in males a confounding finding? *British Journal of Psychiatry, 170,* 234–240.

Jarman, B., Hirsch, S., White, P., & Driscoll, R. (1992). Predicting psychiatric admission rates. *British Medical Journal, 304,* 1146–1151.

Johnstone, E., Crow, T., Johnson, A., & Macmillan, F. (1986). The Northwick Park study of first episodes of schizophrenia. 1: Presentation of the illness and problems relating to admission. *British Journal of Psychiatry, 149,* 51–56.

Johnstone, E., Leary, J., Frith, C., & Owens, D. (1991). Disabilities and circumstances of schizophrenic patients: A follow-up study. VII. Police contact. *British Journal of Psychiatry, 159,* (Suppl. 13), 37–39.

Jones, P.B., Bebbington, P., Foerster, A., Lewis, S., Murray, R., Russel, A., Sham, P., Toone, B., & Wilkins, S. (1993). Premorbid social underachievement in schizophrenia. Results from the Camberwell Collaborative Psychosis Study. *British Journal of Psychiatry, 162*, 65–71.

Jones, P., Rodgers, B., Murray, R., & Marmot, M. (1994a). Child developmental risk factors for adult schizophrenia in the British 1946 birth cohort. *Lancet, 344*, 1398–402.

Jones, P., Harvey, I., Lewis, S., Toone, B., Van Os, J., Williams, M., & Murray, R.M. (1994b). Cerebral ventricle dimensions as risk factors for the functional psychoses. *Psychological Medicine, 24*, 995–1011.

Joyce, P.R. (1987). Changing trends in first admissions and readmissions for mania and schizophrenia in New Zealand. *Australia and New Zealand Journal of Psychiatry, 21*, 82–86.

Kasanin, J. (1933). The acute schizoaffective psychoses. *American Journal of Psychiatry, 13*, 97–126.

Kay, D.W.K., & Roth, M. (1961). Environmental and hereditary factors in the schizophrenias of old age ("late paraphrenia") and their bearing on the general problem of causation in schizophrenia. *Journal of Mental Science, 107*, 649–686.

Kay, D.W.K., Beamish, P., & Roth, M. (1964). Old age mental disorders in Newcastle Upon Tyne. *British Journal of Psychiatry, 110*, 146–158.

Keefe, R.S.E., Frescka, E., Apter, S.H., Davidson, M., Macaluso, J.M., Hirschowitz, J., & Davis, K.L. (1996). Clinical characteristics of Kraepelinian schizophrenia: Replication and extension of previous findings. *American Journal of Psychiatry, 153*, 806–811.

Keith, S.J., Regier, D.A., & Rae, D.S. (1991). Schizophrenic disorders. In L.N. Robins & D.A. Regier (Eds.), *Psychiatric disorders in America*. New York: Free Press.

Kendell, R., Malcolm, D., & Adams, W. (1993). The problem of detecting changes in the incidence of schizophrenia. *British Journal of Psychiatry, 162*, 212–218.

Kendell, R.E., & Zealley, A.K. (1993). Diagnosis and classification. In *Companion to psychiatric studies* (fifth edn). London: Churchill Livingstone.

Kendler, K., Gruenberg, A.M., & Tsuang, M.T. (1985). Psychiatric illness in first-degree relatives of schizophrenic and surgical control patients: A family study using DSM-III criteria. *Archives of General Psychiatry, 42*, 770–779.

Kendler, K., Gruenberg, A.M., & Tsuang, M.T. (1986). A DSM-III family study of the non-schizophrenic psychotic disorders. *American Journal of Psychiatry, 143*, 1098-1105.

Kendler, K.S., & Hays, P. (1983). Schizophrenia subdivided by family history of affective disorder: A comparison of symptomatology and course of illness. *Archives of General Psychiatry, 40*, 951–955.

Kendler, K.S., McGuire, M., Gruenberg, A.M., O'Hare, A., Spellman, M., & Walsh, D. (1993). The Roscommon family study. I. Methods, diagnosis of probands, and risk of schizophrenia in relatives. *Archives of General Psychiatry, 50*, 527–540.

Kety, S.S. (1980). The syndrome of schizophrenia. *British Journal of Psychiatry, 136*, 421–436.

Khoury, M., Beatty, T., & Cohen, B. (1993.) *Fundamentals of genetic epidemiology*. Oxford: Oxford University Press.

Kimura, D. (1992). Sex differences in the brain. *Scientific American, 267*, 81–87.

King, M., Coker, E., Leavey, G., Hoare, A., & Johnson-Sabine, E. (1994). Incidence of psychotic illness in London: Comparison of ethnic groups. *British Medical Journal, 309*, 1115–1119.

Klassen, D., & O'Connor. W. (1988). Crime, inpatient admissions and violence among male mental patients. *International Journal of Law and Psychiatry, 11*, 305–312.

Kleinman, A. (1977). Depression, somatisation and the new "cross cultural" psychiatry. *Social Science Medicine, 11*, 3–10.

Kolle, K. (1931). *Dir primare veruckteit (Primary madness or paranoia)*. Theime: Leipzig.

Kraepelin, E. (1896). *Psychiatrie: Ein Lehrbuch fur Studirende und Aertze.* Leipzig: Barth.

Landau, S. (1981). Juveniles and the police. *British Journal of Criminology, 21,* 27–46.

Lazarsfeld, P.L., & Henry, N.W. (1968). *Latent structure analysis.* Boston, MA: Houghton Mifflin.

Lee, A.S. & Murray, R.M. (1988). The long-term outcome of the Maudsley depressives. *British Journal of Psychiatry, 153,* 741–751.

Leff, J., Fisher, M., & Bertelsen, A. (1976). A cross national study of mania. *British Journal of Psychiatry, 129,* 428–42.

Lewine, R.J. (1988). Gender and schizophrenia. In H.A. Nasrallah (Ed.), *Handbook of schizophrenia,* vol 3. Amsterdam: Elsevier.

Lewis, S.W., & Murray, R.M. (1987). Obstetric complications, neurodevelopmental deviance, and risk of schizophrenia. *Journal of Psychiatric Research, 21,* 413–421.

Lewis, S.W., Owen, M.J., & Murray, R.M. (1989). Obstretric complications and schizophrenia; methodology and mechanisms. In S.C. Schulz & C.A. Tamminga (Eds.), *Schizophrenia: A scientific focus.* New York: Oxford University Press

Lewis, G., Croft-Jeffreys, C., & David, A. (1990). Are British psychiatrists racist? *British Journal Psychiatry, 157,* 410–415.

Lewis, G., David, A., Andréason, S., & Allebeck, P. (1992). Schizophrenia and city life. *Lancet, 340,* 137–140.

Lieberman, J., Jody, D., Geisler, S., Alvir, J., Loebel, A., Szymanski, S., Woerner, M., & Borenstein, M. (1993). Time course and biologic correlates of treatment response in first-episode schizophrenia. *Archives of General Psychiatry, 50,* 369–376.

Lindqvist, P., & Allebeck P. (1990). Schizophrenia and crime: A longitudinal follow up of 644 schizophrenics in Stockholm. *British Journal of Psychiatry, 157,* 345–350.

Link, B., Andrews, H., & Cullen, F. (1992). The violent and illegal behaviour of mental patients reconsidered. *American Sociological Review, 57,* 275–292.

Littlewood, R., & Lipsedge, M. (1982). *Aliens and alienists: Ethnic minorities and psychiatry.* Harmondsworth: Penguin.

Littlewood, R., & Lipsedge, M. (1988). Psychiatric illness among British Afro-Caribbeans. *British Medical Journal, 296,* 950–951.

Loranger, A.W. (1984). Sex differences in age at onset of schizophrenia. *Archives of General Psychiatry, 41,* 157–161.

Luck, D. (1966). Poliomyelitis in Jamaica: A short history with comments upon the effects of immunization. *West Indies Medical Journal, 15,* 189–196.

Mackay, R., & Wight, R. (1984). Schizophrenia and anti-social (criminal) behaviour: Some responses from sufferers and relatives. *Medicine, Science and Law, 24,* 192–198.

MacMillan, J., & Johnson, A. (1987). Contact with the police in early schizophrenia: Its nature, frequency and relevance to the outcome of treatment. *Medicine Science and Law, 27,* 191–200.

Maj, M., & Perris, C. (1990). Patterns of course in patients with a cross-sectional diagnosis of schizoaffective disorder. *Journal of Affective Disorders, 20,* 71–77.

Makanjuola, R.O. (1985). Recurrent unipolar manic disorder in the Yoruba Nigerian: Further evidence. *British Journal of Psychiatry, 147,* 434–437.

Malla, A., Cortese, L., Shaw, T.S., & Ginsberg, B. (1990). Life events and relapse in schizophrenia: A one year prospective study. *Social Psychiatry and Psychiatric Epidemiology, 25,* 221–224.

Marneros, A. Deister, A., Rohde, A., Steinmeyer, E.M., & Junemann, H. (1989). Long-term outcome of schizoaffective and schizophrenic disorders: A comparative study. *European Archives of Psychiatry and Neurological Sciences, 238,* 118–125.

Marneros, A. Deister, A., & Rohde, A. (1990). Psychopathological and social status of patients with affective, schizophrenic and schizoaffective disorders aftyer long-term course. *Acta Psychiatrica Scandinavica, 82*, 352–358.

Marzuk, P. (1996). Violence, crime and mental illness: How strong a link? *Archives of General Psychiatry, 53*, 481–486.

Mayer, W. (1921). Uber paraphrene psychosen. *Zeitsch Gesamte Neurol. Psychiat., 71*, 187–206.

McGlashan, T. (1984). The Chestnut Lodge follow-up study I. Follow-up methodology and study sample. *Archives of General Psychiatry, 41*, 573–585.

McGlashan, T. (1986). Predictors of shorter-, medium- and longer-term outcome in schizophrenia. *American Journal of Psychiatry, 143*, 50–55.

McGorry, P.D., Edwards, J., Mihalopoulos, C., Harrigan, S.M., & Jackson, H.J. (1996). EPPIC: An involving system of early detection and optimal management. *Schizophrenia Bulletin, 22*, 305–326.

McGovern, D., & Cope, R. (1987). First psychiatric admission rates of first and second generation Afro Caribbeans. *Social Psychiatry, 22*, 139–149.

McGovern, D., Hemmings, P., Cope, R., & Lowerson, A. (1994). Long-term follow-up of young Afro-Caribbean Britons and white Britons with a first admission diagnosis of schizophrenia. *Social Psychiatry and Psychiatric Epidemiology, 29*, 8–19.

McGrath, J., & Castle, D.J. (1995). Does influenza cause schizophrenia? A five-year review. *Australian and New Zealand Journal of Psychiatry, 29*, 23–31.

McGuffin, P., Farmer, A.E., & Harvey, I. (1991). A polydiagnostic application of operational criteria in studies of psychotic illness: Development and reliability of the OPCRIT system. *Archives of General Psychiatry, 48*, 764–770.

McGuire, P.K., Jones, P., Harvey, I., Williams, M., McGuffin, P., & Murray, R.M. (1995). Morbid risk of schizophrenia for relatives of patients with cannabis-associated psychosis. *Schizophrenia Research, 15*, 277–281.

McKenzie, K.J., & Crowcroft, N.S. (1994). Race, ethnicity, culture, and science. *British Medical Journal, 309*, 286–87.

McKenzie, K., Van Os, J., Fahy, T., Jones, P., Harvey, I., Toone, B., & Murray, R. (1995). Psychosis with good prognosis in Afro-Caribbean people now living in the United Kingdom. *British Medical Journal, 311*, 1325–1328.

Modestin, J., & Ammann, R. (1996). Mental disorder and criminality: Male schizophrenia. *Schizophrenia Bulletin, 22*, 69–82.

Munk-Jørgensen, P. (1986). Decreasing first-admission rates of schizophrenia among males in Denmark from 1970 to 1984. Changing diagnostic patterns? *Acta Psychiatrica Scandinavica, 73*, 645–50.

Munk-Jørgensen, P., & Mortensen, P. (1993). Incidence and epidemiology of schizophrenia in Denmark. *British Journal of Psychiatry, 162*, 268–269.

Munro, A. (1988). Delusional (paranoid) disorders: Etiologic and taxonomic considerations. *Canadian Journal of Psychiatry, 33*, 171–174.

Munro, A. (1991). A plea for paraphrenia. *Canadian Journal of Psychiatry, 36*, 667–672.

Murray, R.M., Lewis, S.W., & Reveley, A.M. (1985). Towards an aetiological classification of schizophrenia. *Lancet, i*, 1023–1026.

Murray, R.M., & O'Callaghan, E. (1991). The congenital and adult-onset psychoses: Kraepelin lost, Kraepelin found. In A. Kerr & H. McClelland (Eds.), *Concepts of mental disorder: A continuing debate* (pp. 48–65). London: Gaskell.

Murray, R.M., O'Callaghan, E., Castle, D.J., & Lewis, S.W. (1992). A neurodevelopmental approach to the classification of schizophrenia. *Schizophrenia Bulletin, 18*, 319–332.

Murphy, D.G.M., DeCarli, C., McIntosh, A.R., Daly, E., Mentis, M.J., Pietrini, P., Szczepanik, J., Schapiro, M.B., Grady, C.L., Horwitz, B., & Papoport, S.I. (1996). Sex differences in human brain morphometry and metabolism: An invivo quantitative magnetic resonance imaging and positron emission tomograph study on the effect of aging. *Archives of General Psychiatry, 53,* 585–594.

Navarro, F., Van Os, J., Jones, P., & Murray, R.M. (1996). Explaining sex differences in course and outcome in the functional psychoses. *Schizophrenia Research, 21,* 161–170.

Neave, H. (1979). *Elementary statistical tables.* London: George Allen.

Nicoll, A., & Logan, S. (1989). Viral infections of pregnancy and childhood. In J. Cruickshank & D.Beevers (Eds.), *Ethnic factors in health and disease.* London: Wright.

O'Callaghan, E., Larkin, C., & Waddington, J.L. (1990). Obstetric complications in schizophrenia and the validity of maternal recall. *Psychological Medicine, 20,* 89–94.

O'Callaghan, E., Sham, P., Takei, N., Glover, G., & Murray, R. (1991). Prenatal exposure to the "Asian Flu" epidemic and later schizophrenia. *Lancet, 337,* 1248–1250.

Opler, L.A., Kay, S.R., Rosado, V., & Lindenmayer, J-P. (1984). Positive and negative syndromes in chronic schizophrenic inpatients. *Journal of Nervous and Mental Disease, 172,* 317–325.

Orel, O., Cannon, T.D., Hollister, J.M., Mednick, S.A.., & Parnas, J. (1991). Ventricular enlargement and premorbid deficits in school-occupational attainment. *Schizophrenia Research, 4,* 49–52.

Owen, M.J., Lewis, S.W., & Murray, R.M. (1989). Family history and cerebral ventricular enlargement in schizophrenia: A case control study. *British Journal of Psychiatry, 154,* 629–634.

Parker, G., O' Donnell, M., & Walters, S. (1985). Changes in the diagnosis of the functional psychoses associated with the introduction of lithium. *British Journal of Psychiatry, 146,* 377–382.

Parsons, P.L. (1964). Mental health of Swansea's old folk. *British Journal of Preventative and Social Medicine, 19,* 43–47.

Parsons, C. (1983). West Indian children with multiple congenital defects. *Archives of Diseases in Childhood, 38,* 454–458.

Paykell, E. (1978). Contribution of life events to causation to psychiatric illness. *Psychological Medicine, 8,* 245–253.

Pearlson, G.D., Garbacz, D.J., Moberg, P.J., Ahn, H.S., & de Paulo, J.R. (1985). Symptomatic, familial, perinatal, and social correlates of computer axial tomography (CAT) changes in schizophrenia and bipolars. *Journal of Nervous and Mental Disease, 173,* 42–50.

Pearlson, G.D., Kim, W.S., Kubos, K.L., Moberg, P.J., Jayaram, G., Bascom, M.J., Chase, G.A., Goldfinger, A.D., & Tune, L.E. (1989). Ventricle–brain ratio, computed tomographic density, and brain area in 50 schizophrenics. *Archives of General Psychiatry, 46,* 690–697.

Pearson, M. (1991). Ethnic differences in infant health. *Archives of Diseases in Childhood, 66,* 88–90.

Philips, L. (1953). Case history data and prognosis in schizophrenia. *Journal of Nervous Mental Disorders, 117,* 515–525.

Post, F. (1966). *Persistent persecutory states of the elderly.* Oxford: Pergamon.

Powell, R.B., Hollander, D., & Tobiansky, R.I. (1995). Crisis in admission beds: A four-year survey of the bed state of Greater London's acute psychiatric units. *British Journal of Psychiatry, 167,* 765–769.

Prince, M.J., & Phelan, M.C. (1990). Trends in schizophrenia. *Lancet, 335,* 851–852.

Rabins, P., Paulker, S., & Thomas, J. (1984). Can schizophrenia begin after age 44? *Comprehensive Psychiatry, 25,* 290–293.

Raleigh, V., & Balarajan, R. (1982). Suicide levels and trends among immigrants in England and Wales. *Health Trends, 24,* 91–94.

Riecher, A., Maurer, K., Loffler, W., Fatkenheuer, B., an der Heiden, W., & Hafner, H. (1989). Schizophrenia: A disease of young single males? *European Archives of Psychiatry and Neurological Sciences, 239,* 210–212.

Riecher-Rossler, A., & Hafner, H. (1993). Schizophrenia and oestrogens: Is there an association? *European Archives of Psychiatry and Clinical Neuroscience, 242,* 323–328.

Rifkin, L., Lewis, S., Jones, P.B., Toone, B.K., & Murray, R.M. (1994). Low birth weight and schizophrenia. *British Journal of Psychiatry, 165,* 353–356.

Robertson, G. (1988). Arrest patterns among mentally disordered offenders. *British Journal of Psychiatry, 153,* 313–316.

Robins, E., & Guze, S.B. (1970). Establishment of diagnostic validity in psychiatric illness: its application to schizophrenia. *American Journal of Psychiatry, 126,* 983–987.

Rogers, B. (1990). Behaviour and personality in childhood as predictors of adult psychiatric disorder. *Journal of Child Psychology and Psychiatry, 3,* 393–414.

Roth, M. (1955). The natural history of mental disorder in old age. *Journal of Mental Science, 101,* 281–301.

Rothman, K. (1986). *Modern epidemiology.* Boston: Little, Brown.

Russell, A.J., Munro, J.C., Jones, P.B., Hemsley, D.R., & Murray, R.M. (1997). Schizophrenia and the myth of intellectual decline. *American Journal of Psychiatry, 154,* 635–639.

Rwegellera, G. (1977). Psychiatric morbidity among West Africans and West Indians living in London. *Psychological Medicine, 7,* 317–329.

Sashidharan, S.P. (1993). Afro-Caribbeans and schizophrenia: The ethnic vulnerability hypothesis re-examined. *International Review of Psychiatry, 5,* 129–144.

Scharfetter, C., & Nusperli, M. (1980). The group of schizophrenias, schizoaffective psychoses and affective disorders. *Schizophrenia Bulletin, 4,* 586–591.

Schlesselman, J. (1982). *Case–control studies: Design, conduct, analysis.* New York: Oxford University Press.

Schneier, F., & Siris, S. (1987). A review of psychoactive substance use and abuse in schizophrenia: Patterns of drug abuse. *Journal of Nervous and Mental Disease 175,* 641–652.

Seeman, M.V. (1986). Current outcome in schizophrenia: Women vs men. *Acta Psychiatrica Scandinavica, 73,* 609–617.

Seeman, M.V. (1989). Prenatal gonadal hormones and schizophrenia in men and women. *Psychiatric Journal of the University of Ottawa, 14,* 473–475.

Selten, J.P., & Sijben, N. (1994). First admission rates for schizophrenia in immigrants to the Netherlands. The Dutch National Register. *Social Psychiatry and Psychiatric Epidemiology, 29,* 71–77.

Sham, P.C., Castle, D.J., Wesseley, S., Farmer, A.E, & Murray, R.M. (1996). Further exploration of a latent class typology of schizophrenia. *Schizophrenia Research, 20,* 105–115.

Sham, P.C., Jones, P., Russel, A., Gilvarry K., Wilkins, S., Foerster, A., Bebbington, P., Lewis, S., Toone, B., & Murray, R. (1994a). Age at onset, sex, and familial psychiatric morbidity in schizophrenia. Report from the Camberwell Collaborative Psychosis Study. *British Journal of Psychiatry 165,* 466–473.

Sham, P.C., MacLean, C.J., & Kendler, K.S. (1994b). A typological model of schizophrenia based on age at onset, sex, and familial morbidity. *Acta Psychiatrica Scandinavica, 89,* 135–141.

Shepherd, M., Watt, D., & Falloon, I. (1989). The natural history of schizophrenia: A five year follow-up study of outcome prediction in a representative sample of schizophrenics. *Psychological Medicine,* monograph supplement 15. Cambridge: Cambridge University Press.

Shimizu, A., Kurachi, M., Noda, M., Yamaguchi, N., Torri, H., & Isaki, K. (1988). Influence of sex on age at onset of schizophrenia. *Japanese Journal of Psychiatry and Neurology, 42*, 35–40.

Siegel, J.S. (1974). Estimates of coverage of the population by sex, race and age in the 1970 census. *Demography, 11*, 1–23.

Smith, D., & Gray, J. (1983). *Police and people in London* (vol. IV): *The police in action.* London: Policy Studies Institute.

Sokal, R. (1988). Genetic, geographic and linguistic distances in Europe. *Proceedings of the National Academy of Sciences of the USA, 85*, 1722–1726.

Sokal, R., Harding, R.M., & Oden, N.L. (1989). Spatial patterns of human gene frequencies in Europe. *American Journal of Physical Anthropology, 80*, 267–294.

Spitzer, R., Endicott, J., & Robins, E. (1978). Research Diagnostic Criteria (RDC): Rationale and reliability. *Archives General Psychiatry, 35*, 773–782.

STATA Corp. (1995). *Stata Statistical Software: Release 4.0.* College Station, TX: STATA Corporation.

Steer, D. (1973). The elusive conviction. *British Journal of Criminology, 13*, 373–83.

Stevens, P., & Willis, C. (1979). *Race, crime and arrests.* Home Office Research Unit Report No 58. London: HMSO.

Stoffelmayr, B., Dillavou, D., & Hunter, J. (1983). Premorbid functioning and outcome in schizophrenia: A cumulative analysis. *Journal of Consulting and Clinical Psychology, 51*, 338–352.

Strauss, J.S., & Carpenter, W.T. (1978). The prognosis of schizophrenia: Rationale for a multidimensional concept. *Schizophrenia Bulletin, 4*, 56–67.

Sugarman, P.A. (1992). Outcome of schizophrenia in the Afro-Caribbean community. Social *Psychiatry & Psychiatric Epidemiology, 27*, 102–5.

Sugarman, P., & Crawford, D. (1994). Schizophrenia in the Afro-Caribbean community. *British Journal of Psychiatry, 164*, 474–480.

Susser, M., & Susser, E. (1987). Separating heredity and environment. I. Genetic and environmental indices. In M. Susser (Ed.), *Epidemiology, health and society: Selected papers.* New York: Oxford University Press.

Swanson, J., Holzer, C., Ganju, V., & Jono, R. (1990). Violence and psychiatric disorder in the community: Evidence from the Epidemiologic Catchment Area Surveys. *Hospital Community Psychiatry, 41*, 761–770.

Takei, N., O'Callaghan, E., Sham, P., Glover, G., Tamura, A., & Murray, R.M. (1992). Seasonality of admissions in the psychoses: Effect of diagnosis, sex, and age at onset. *British Journal of Psychiatry, 161*, 506–511.

Takei, N., Lewis, G., Sham, P.C., & Murray, R.M. (1996). Age–period–cohort analysis of the incidence of schizophrenia in Scotland. *Psychological Medicine, 26*, 963–973.

Tardiff, K., & Sweillam, A. (1980). Assault, suicide and mental illness. *Archives of General Psychiatry, 37*, 164–169.

Taylor, D.C. (1969). Differential rates of cerebral maturation between the sexes and between hemispheres. *Lancet, ii*, 140–142.

Taylor, M. (1992). Are schizophrenia and affective disorder related? A selective literature review. *American Journal of Psychiatry, 149*, 22–32.

Taylor, P. (1985). Motives for offending amongst violent and psychotic men. *British Journal of Psychiatry, 147*, 491–498.

Taylor, P., & Gunn, J. (1984). Violence and psychosis 1: Risk of violence among psychotic men. *British Medical Journal, 288*, 1945–1949.

Taylor, P., Mullen, P., & Wessely, S. (1996). Psychosis, violence and crime. In J. Gunn, & P. Taylor (Eds.), *Forensic psychiatry: Clinical, ethical and legal issues.* London: Heinemann.

Teague, A. (1993). Ethnic group: First results from the 1991 census. *Population Trends, 72,* 12–17.

Terry, O., Condie, R., Bissenden, J., & Kerridge, D. (1987). Ethnic differences in incidence of very low birth weight and neonatal deaths among normally formed infants. *Archives of Diseases in Childhood, 62,* 709–711.

Torrey, E.F., & Bowler, A. (1991). Geographical distribution of insanity in America: Evidence for an urban factor. *Schizophrenia Bulletin, 16,* 591–604.

Townsend, P., Phillimore, P., & Beattie, A. (1988). *Health and deprivation: Inequality and the North.* London: Croom-Helm.

Tsuang, M.T., & Winoker, G. (1974). Criteria for subtyping schizophrenia: Clinical differentiation of hebephrenic and paranoid schizophrenia. *Archives of General Psychiatry, 31,* 43–47.

Tsuang, M.T., & Dempsey, G.M. (1979). Long term outcome of major psychoses II. Schizoaffective disorder, compared with schizophrenia, affective disorders, and a surgical control group. *Archives of General Psychiatry, 36,* 1302–1304.

Tsuang, M., Winokur, G., & Crowe, R.R. (1980). Morbid risks of schizophrenia and affective disorders among first degree relatives of patients with schizophrenia, mania, depression, and surgical conditions. *British Journal of Psychiatry, 137,* 497–504.

Vaillant, G.E. (1964). Prospective prediction of schizophrenic remission. *Archives of General Psychiatry, 11,* 509–518.

Vallès, V., Guillamat, R., Fañanas, L., Gutiérrez, B., Campillo, M., & Van Os, J. (1996). Increased morbid risk of schizophrenia in relatives of patients with severe bipolar disorder. *European Psychiatry, 11* (suppl 4), 306s–307s.

Van Os, J. (1995). *(Genetic) Epidemiology as a tool to examine risk factors for onset and persistence of illness in the functional psychoses.* Mastricht: Mastricht University Press

Van Os, J., Castle, D., Takei, N., Der, G., & Murray, R. (1996a). Psychotic illness in ethnic minorities: Clarification from the 1991 census. *Psychological Medicine, 26,* 203–208.

Van Os, J., Fahy, T., Bebbington, P., Wilkins, S., Jones, P., Gilvarry, K., Lewis, S., Toone, B., & Murray, R. (1994). The influence of life events on the subsequent course of psychotic illness: A follow-up of the Camberwell Collaborative Psychosis study. *Psychological Medicine, 24,* 503–513

Van Os, J., Fahy, T., Jones, P., Harvey, I., Lewis, S., Williams, M., Toone, B., & Murray, R. (1995). Increased intra-cerebral CSF spaces predict unemployment and negative symptoms in psychotic illness: A prospective study. *British Journal of Psychiatry, 166,* 750–759.

Van Os, J., Fahy, T., Jones, P., Harvey, I., Lewis, S., Sham, P., Toone, B., & Murray, R. (1996b). Psychopathological syndromes in the functional psychoses: Associations with course and outcome. *Psychological Medicine, 26,* 203–208.

Van Os, J., Galdos, P., Lewis, G., Mann, M., & Bourgeois, M. (1993). Schizophrenia sans frontières. *British Medical Journal, 307,* 489–492

Van Os, J., Jones, P. Lewis, G., Wadsworth, M., & Murray, R.M. (1997a). Developmental precursors of affective illness in a general population birth cohort. *Archives of General Psychiatry, 54,* 625–631.

Van Os, J., Marcelis, M., Sham, P., Jones, P., Gilvarry, K., & Murray, R. (1997b). Psychopathological syndromes and familial morbid risk of psychosis. *British Journal of Psychiatry, 170,* 241–246.

Van Os, J., Takei, N., Castle, D., Wessely, S., Der, G., & Murray, R. (1996c). Premorbid abnormalities in mania, schizophrenia, acute schizomania and chronic schizophrenia. *Social Psychiatry & Psychiatric Epidemiology, 30,* 274–279.

Van Os, J., Takei, N., Castle, D., & Murray, R.M. (1996d). The incidence of mania: Time trends in relation to gender and ethnic group. *Social Psychiatry & Psychiatric Epidemiology, 31,* 129–136.

Ventura, J., Nuechterlein, K.H., Lukoff, D., & Hardisty, J.P. (1989). A prospective study of stressful life events and schizophrenic relapse. *Journal of Abnormal Psychology, 98*, 407–411.

Verdoux, H., Van Os, J., Sham, P., Jones, P., Gilvarry, K., & Murray, R. (1996). Does famiality predict both onset and persistence of illness in the functional psychoses? A prospective study. *British Journal of Psychiatry, 168*, 620–626.

Verdoux, M., Geddes, J.R., Takei, N., Bovet, P., Eagles, J.M., Heun, R., McCready, R., McNeill, T., O'Callaghan, E., Strober, G., Willinger, M., Wright, P., & Murray, R.M. (1997). Obstetric complication and age at onset in schizophrenia: An international collaborative meta analysis of individual patient data. *American Journal of Psychiatry, 154*, 1220–1227.

Waddington, J.L., & Youssef, H.A. (1994). Evidence for a gender-specific decline in the rate of schizophrenia in rural Ireland over a 50-year period. *British Journal of Psychiatry, 164*, 171–6.

Walker, G., Ashley, D., McCraw, A., & Bernard, G. (1986). Maternal mortality in Jamaica. *Lancet, i*, 486–488.

Weinberger, D.R., Cannon-Spoor, E., Potkin, S.G., & Wyatt, R.J. (1980). Poor premorbid adjustment and CT scan abnormalities in chronic schizophrenia. *American Journal of Psychiatry, 137*, 1410–1413.

Weinberger, D.R., DeLisi, L.E., Perman, G.P., Targum, S., & Wyatt, R.J. (1982). Computed tomography in schizophreniform disorder and other acute psychiatric disorders. *Archives of General Psychiatry, 39*, 778–783.

Werry, J.S., McClellan, J.M., & Chard, L. (1991). Childhood and adolescent schizophrenic, bipolar, and schizoaffective disorders: A clinical and outcome study. *Journal of the American Academy of Child and Adolescent Psychiatry, 30*, 457–465.

Wessely, S. (1994). *The criminal careers of incidence cases of schizophrenia.* MD thesis, University of London.

Wessely, S., Castle, D., Der, G., & Murray, R. (1991). Schizophrenia and Afro-Caribbeans: A case–control study. *British Journal of Psychiatry, 159*, 795–801.

Wessely, S., & Castle, D. (1992). How valid are case notes for assessing criminal history? *Journal of Forensic Psychiatry, 3*, 359–363.

Wessely, S., & Taylor, P. (1991). Madness and crime; criminology or psychiatry? *Criminal Behaviour and Mental Health, 1*, 193–228.

Wessely, S., Castle, D., Douglas, A., & Taylor, P. (1994). The criminal careers of incident cases of schizophrenia. *Psychological Medicine, 24*, 483–502.

West, D., & Farrington, D. (1973). *Who becomes delinquent?* London: Heinemann.

Williamson, J., Stokoe, I.H., Gray, S., Fisher, M., & Smith, A. (1964). Old people at home: Their unreported needs. *Lancet, i*, 1117–1120.

Wing, L. (1979). Mentally retarded children in Camberwell, London. In H. Hafner (Ed.), *Estimating needs for mental health care.* New York: Springer-Verlag.

Wing, J.K., & Hailey, A.M. (1972). *Evaluating a community psychiatric service: The Camberwell register, 1964–1971.* London: Oxford University Press.

Wing, J.K., Cooper, J.E., & Sartorius, N. (1974). *The measurement and classification of psychiatric symptoms.* Cambridge: Cambridge University Press.

Woodruff, P., & Murray, R.M. (1994). The aetiology of brain abnormalities in schizophrenia. In Ed R. Ancill (Ed.), *Schizophrenia: Exploring the spectrum of psychoses.* New York: Wiley.

World Health Organisation. (1978). *Mental disorders: Glossary and guide to their classification in accordance with the ninth revision of the International Classification of Diseases (ICD-9).* Geneva: WHO.

World Health Organisation. (1993). *The ICD-10 classification of mental and behavioural disorders: Clinical descriptions and diagnostic guidelines.* Geneva: WHO.

GLOSSARY

APA: American Psychiatric Association

CATEGO: Computer programme for PSE

CRO: Criminal Records Office (England and Wales)

CT: computerised tomography

DF: degrees of freedom

DSM: Diagnostic and Statistical Manual (of the American Psychiatric Association)

EGRET: statistical software for regression

FH-RDC: family history schedule for Research Diagnostic Criteria

HR: hazard ratio

ICD: International Classification of Disease (of the World Health Organisation)

LRS: likelihood ratio statistic

M-H: Mantel–Haenzel (test for linear trend)

MLLSA: Maximum likelihood latent structure analysis

N: number

NIMH: National Institute of Mental Health (US)

95% CI: 95% confidence interval

OC: obstetric (pregnancy or birth) complication

OR: odds ratio

OCCPI: Operational Criteria Checklist for Psychotic Illness

OPCRIT: computer programme for OCCPI

OPCS: Office for Population Censuses and Surveys (UK)

PSE: Present State Examination

RDC: Research Diagnostic Criteria

RR: rate ratio or risk ratio

SD: standard deviation

SKUMIX: statistical software for assessment of distributions

UK: United Kingdom

US: United States of America

VBR: ventricle:brain ratio

WHO: World Health Organisation

Appendix 1a. Data collection sheets for Camberwell register study: General

Camberwell Register Schizophrenia Project

Note: if data unknown, score 9

Register Number:	☐☐☐☐☐☐
Hospital Number:	☐☐☐☐☐☐
Age of patient at contact (yrs):	☐☐
dob (day month year):	☐☐☐☐☐☐
inpatient (no = 0; yes = 1)	☐
Occupation of father (nil = 0; manual = 1; white collar = 2; professional = 3)	
Ethnicity (Caucasion = 0; African-Carribean = 1; African = 2; Asian = 3; other = 4)	
patient	☐
father	☐
mother	☐
Country of birth (UK & Eire = 0; W Indies = 1; Africa = 2; Asia = 3; other = 4)	
patient	☐
father	☐
mother	☐

Age of patient entry to UK (yrs) (if applicable)   □□
Criminality of parents (conviction only) (no = 0; yes = 1)
   father   □
   mother   □
Alcohol problem in parents (no = 0; yes = 1)
   father   □
   mother   □
Obstetric complications (code a separate scale)   □
Developmental problems (code as separate scale)
   developmental score   □
Childhood neurotical traits (no = 0; yes = 1)
   enuresis   □
   nailbiting   □
   school refusal   □
Child care (not applicable = 0; poor = 1; good = 2)   □
   (rate poor if: malnutrition, neglect, or social service
   involvement)
Academic achievement (no exams = 0; CSE = 1; O-level = 2;   □
   A-level = 3, 3o = 4)
Criminality (no = 0; yes = 1)   □
   (include: juvenile offences, juvenile cautions, adult arrest,
   conviction)
Juvenile delinquency (no = 0; yes = 1)   □
   (include: drugs, arrest, expelled, truant, stealing,
   vandal, runaway, arson)
Premorbid employment (not on job market = 0;   □
   unstable = 3 or more in 5 yrs = 1; unemployed = 6 or more
   months last 5 yrs = 2; stable = 3)
Premorbid sexual/marital adjustment
   married or living as (no = 0; yes = 1)   □
   marital violence (physical only) (no = 0; yes = 1)   □
   marital desertion (no = 0; yes = 1)   □
   more than 10 sexual contacts per year (no = 0; yes = 1)   □
   no relationships (no = 0; yes = 1)   □
   first sex before 14 years (no = 0; yes = 1)   □
Drug problem (no = 0; recreational = 1; problem = 2)
   alcohol   □
   cannabis   □
   heroin   □
   other   □
Violence on admission (no = 0; yes = 1)
   police involvement   □
   violent to self   □

violent to others ☐
Inpatient aggression (no = 0; yes = 1) ☐
Delusional behaviour (no = 0; yes = 1) ☐
Evidence of organicity (no = 0; yes = 1)
   EEG abnormal ☐
   CT scan abnormal ☐
Homeless on discharge (no = 0; yes = 1) ☐
Outpatient contact (no = 0; yes = 1) ☐

Appendix 1B
Data collection sheets for Camberwell register study: Developmental scale

RATING SCALE FOR DEVELOPMENTAL PROBLEMS

SPEECH ☐

0– No problems reported by mother
1– No talk other than mama or dada by age 3. Speech problems still exist at school entry. Either grammar or pronounciation faulty.
2– As above but professional help sought or child referred to educational psychologist or speech therapist by school.

MOTOR ☐

0– No problems reported by mother
1– Could not walk unsupported before 2 years
2– As above but professional advice sought

ENCOPRESIS ☐

0– No problems reported by mother
1– Soiling after age 4 at least once a week over a period of at least 6 weeks
2– As above but professional help sought and physical cause excluded

ENURESIS □

0– No problems reported by mother
1– Bed wetting or day time wetting continuously beyond the age of 5 at least once a week
2– Professional help sought. Physical causes excluded

READING DIFFICULTIES □

0– No problems learning to read or spell
1– Reading or spelling difficulties reported by mother
2– Remedial teaching for reading and spelling required but no special schooling

DEVELOPMENTAL SCORE □

0– No problems reported by mother in any area
1– Problems reported by mother in one or more areas but no professional advice sought
2– Professional advice sought by mother or referral to EP or speech therapist by school for at least one of the above

Appendix 1C
Data collection sheets for Camberwell register study: Obstetric complications scale

OBSTETRIC COMPLICATIONS SCALE:
RATING SCALE FOR DEVELOPMENTAL PROBLEMS

Score: Definite = 2
        Equivocal = 1
        Absent = 0
        Insufficient information = 9

Antepartum:

(Equivocal: ☐
    pre-eclampsia NOS)

1. Rubella or syphilis   ☐
2. Rhesus incompatability   ☐
3. Pre-eclampsia: severe and/or leading to early induction or   ☐
   hospitalisation
4. APH or threatended abortion   ☐

Intrapartum:

(Equivocal: ☐
    Labour >24 or "long/difficult/precipitate" NOS
    Twin birth NOS
    Cord knotted or round neck
    "premature" or "postmature" NOS
    Caesarian NOS
    Forceps or other instrumental delivery, NOS
    <5 1/2 ib (2500g) or "small" NOS
    Incubator/resuscitation/"blue" NOS
    Gross physical anomaly)

5. Premature rupture of membranes, >24 hours   ☐
6. Labour >36 hours or < 3 hours   ☐
7. Twin birth, complicated   ☐
8. Cord prolapse   ☐
9. Gestational age <37 weeks or >42 weeks   ☐
10. Caesarian, complicated or emergency   ☐
11. Breech or abnormal presentation   ☐
12. High or "difficult" forceps   ☐
13. Birthweight <4 1/2 lbs (2000g)   ☐
14. Incubator >4 weeks   ☐

This scale represents a consensus derived from six scales previously used, three from the obstetric and three from the psychiatric literature:

Hobel et al. (1973). *Am. J. Obstetr. Gynae.*
Prechtel et al. (1967). *Br. Med. Journ.*
Littman & Parmalee (1978). *Pediatrics.*
Woerner et al. (1973). *Acta Psychiat. Scand.*
Zax et al. (1977). *Am. J. Orthopsychiat.*
Parnas et al. (1982). *Brit. J. Psychiatr.*

(Four of these are reviewed and compared in Molfese & Thomson (1985), *Chld Dev*).

All items on the derived scale are complications appearing in agreement in at least three of the six scales. Maternal non-pregnancy variables such as age, parity, and history of previous abortion were not included. A few notes on scoring:

1. "Equivocal" complications are counted as present if the listed conditions are met or if one of the definite complications is

"probably" present. This latter condition requires conservative discretion on the part of the scorer.

2. Complications are not additive. If more than one definite complication is present, the item is still scored as "2". Likewise, if more than one equivocal complication is present, the item is still scored as "1".

3. It should be noted that some "complications" such as induction or jaundice should not be scored, since they are of high incidence and of doubtful significance.

Appendix 1D
Data collection sheets for Camberwell register study: OCCPI 2.5

ID Number		☐☐☐☐	
1.	Sex code (0,1)	☐	5
2,3.	Age of onset	☐☐	6,7
4.	Single (0,1)	☐	8
5.	Unemployed (0,1)	☐	9
6.	Duration of illness at least 2 weeks (0,1)	☐	10
7.	Duration of illness at least 6 months (0,1)	☐	11
8.	Duration of prodromal/acute/residual stages at least six months (0,1)	☐	12
9.	Poor premorbid work adjustment (0,1)	☐	13
10.	Poor premorbid social adjustment (0,1)	☐	14
11.	Premorbid personality disorder (0,1)	☐	15
12.	Alcohol/drug abuse within on year of onset (0,1)	☐	16
13.	Family history of schizophrenia (0,1)	☐	17
14.	Family history of other psychiatric disorder (0,1)	☐	18
15.	Bizarre behaviour (0,1)	☐	19
16.	Catatonia (0,1)	☐	20
17.	Speech difficult to understand (0,1)	☐	21
18.	Incoherent (0,1)	☐	22
19.	Positive formal thought disorder	☐	23
20.	Negative formal thought disorder (0,1)	☐	24
21.	Affective symptoms predominate (0,1)	☐	25
22.	Restricted affect (0,1)	☐	26

23.	Blunted affect (0,1)	☐ 27
24.	Inappropriate affect (0,1)	☐ 28
25.	Rapport difficult (0,1)	☐ 29
26.	Persecutory delusions (0,1)	☐ 30
27.	Well-organised delusions (0,1)	☐ 31
28.	Grandiose delusions (0–2)	☐ 32
29.	Delusions of influence (0,1)	☐ 33
30.	Bizarre delusions (0,1)	☐ 34
31.	Widespread delusions (0,1)	☐ 35
32.	Delusions of passivity (0–2)	☐ 36
33.	Primary delusional perception (0–2)	☐ 37
34.	Other primary delusions (0,1)	☐ 38
35.	Delusions and hallucinations lasting one week (0,1)	☐ 39
36.	Persecutory/jealous delusions with hallucinations (0,1)	☐ 40
37.	Thought insertion (0–2)	☐ 41
38.	Thought withdrawal (0–2)	☐ 42
39.	Thought broadcast (0–2)	☐ 43
40.	Thought echo (0–2)	☐ 44
41.	Third person auditory hallucinations (0–2)	☐ 45
42.	Running commentary voices (0–2)	☐ 46
43.	Abusive/accusatory/persecutory voices (0,1)	☐ 47
44.	Other (non affective) auditory hallucinations (0,1)	☐ 48
45.	Information not credible (0,1)	☐ 49
46.	Lack of insight (0,1)	☐ 50
47.	Deterioration from premorbid level of functioning (0,1)	☐ 51
48.	Schizophrenic symptoms respond to neuroleptics (0,1)	☐ 52
49.	Non-affective hallucination in any modality (0,1)	☐ 53
50.	Elevated mood (0–2)	☐ 54
51.	Irritable mood (0–2)	☐ 55
52.	Schizophrenic symptoms at some time as affective symptoms (0,1)	☐ 56
53.	Excessive activity (0–2)	☐ 57
54.	Reckless activity (0–2)	☐ 58
55.	Pressured speech (0–2)	☐ 59
56.	Increased self esteem (0–2)	☐ 60
57.	Thought racing (0–2)	☐ 61
58.	Distractibility (0–2)	☐ 62
59.	Reduced need for sleep (0–2)	☐ 63
60.	Dysphoria (0–3)	☐ 64
61.	Agitated activity (0–3)	☐ 65
62.	Slowed activity (0–3)	☐ 66
63.	Loss of energy/tiredness (0–3)	☐ 67
64.	Loss of pleasure (0–3)	☐ 68

65.	Poor concentration (0–3)	☐ 69
66.	Excessive self-reproach (0–3)	☐ 70
67.	Suicidal ideation (0–3)	☐ 71
68.	Initial insomnia (0–3)	☐ 72
69.	Early morning waking (0–3)	☐ 73
70.	Excessive sleep (0–3)	☐ 74
71.	Poor appetite (0–3)	☐ 75
72.	Weight loss (0–3)	☐ 76
73.	Increased appetite (0–3)	☐ 77
74.	Weight gain (0–3)	☐ 78

Appendix 2
Glossary for rating items in OCCPI 2.5

GLOSSARY FOR OPERATIONAL CRITERIA
CHECKLIST FOR PSYCHOTIC ILLNESS (OCCPI)
(OPCRIT VERSION 2.5)

Specification of items

Following the general approach adopted by the authors of the Present State Examination (PSE), we have produced a glossary to be used with the OPCRIT checklist that provides definitions of every item. This can be referred to in written form when completing a checklist. Alternatively, when entering the data directly onto computer using the OPCRIT programs, a "Help" facility can be called that displays the definition of each item on the screen. The specification of items, where possible, follows the descriptions provided by authors of the various criteria. Otherwise the definitions of signs and symptoms follows the description in standard textbooks and takes as a model the glossary of the PSE.

The definition and coding of each item follow:

1. Sex code: 0 indicates male; 1, female.
2,3. Age at onset: This should be given to the nearest year and is defined as the earliest age at which medical advice was sought for psychiatric reasons or at which symptoms began to cause subjective distress or impair functioning (enter age in years, e.g. 35).

4. Single: The patient has never married or lived as married (0 indicates married; 1, single).

5. Unemployed: The patient was not employed at onset as defined above. Women working full-time in the home are scored as if employed. Students attending classes on full-time course are scored as if employed (0, employed; 1, unemployed).

6. Duration of illness at least 2 weeks: Persistent symptoms or disability such that the patient did not return to premorbid level of functioning within 2 weeks (0, 1 [illness lasted 2 weeks]).

7. Duration of illness at least 6 months: Persistent symptoms or disability such that the patient did not return to premorbid level of functioning within 6 months (0, 1 [illness lasted 6 months]).

8. Duration of total prodromal/acute and residual stages at least 6 months: Total duration of illness is 6 months when prodromal and residual disabilities are included with the acute phase of illness. Prodromal/residual phase symptoms (any two of the following before or after the acute episode): social isolation/marked impairment in role/markedly peculiar behaviour/marked impairment in personal hygiene/blunted, flat, or inappropriate affect/digressive, vague, over-elaborate speech/odd or bizarre ideation/unusual perceptual experiences (0,1 [illness lasted 6 months]).

9. Poor work adjustment: This refers to work history before onset of illness. It should be scored if the patient was unable to keep any job for more than 6 months, had a history of frequent changes of job, or was only able to sustain a job well below that expected by his or her educational level or training at the time of first psychiatric contact. Also score positively for a persistently very poor standard of housework (homemakers) and badly failing to keep up with studies (students) (0, absent; 1, poor work adjustment).

10. Poor premorbid social adjustment: Patient found difficulty entering or maintaining normal social relationships, showed persistent social isolation or withdrawal, or maintained solitary interests before onset of psychotic symptoms (0, absent; 1, poor social adjustment).

11. Premorbid personality disorder: Evidence of inadequate/schizoid/schizotypal/paranoid/ cyclothymic/psychopathic/sociopathic personality disorder present since adolescence and before onset of psychotic symptoms (0, absent; 1, personality disorder present).

12. Alcohol/other drug abuse within 1 year of onset of psychotic symptoms: alcohol abuse where quantity is excessive (rater judgement) where alcohol-related complications occur, during the year before first psychiatric contact (rated strictly as exclusion criteria for some definitions of schizophrenia); other drug abuse where non prescribed drugs are repeatedly taken or prescribed drugs are used in

excessive quantities and without medical supervision in the year before first psychiatric contact (0, absent; 1, family history present).

13. Family history of schizophrenia: Definite history of schizophrenia in a first or second-degree relative (0, absent; 1, family history present).

14. Family history of other psychiatric disorder: First or second-degree relative has another psychiatric disorder severe enough to warrant psychiatric referral (0, absent; 1, family history present).

15. Bizarre behaviour: Behaviour that is strange and incomprehensible to others; includes behaviour that could be interpreted as a response to auditory hallucinations or thought interference (0, absent; 1, present).

16. Catatonia: Patient exhibits persistent mannerisms, stereotypes, posturing, catalepsy, stupor, or excitement that is not explicable by affective change (0, absent; 1, present).

17. Speech difficult to understand: Speech that makes communication difficult because of lack of logical or understandable organisation; does not include dysarthria or speech impediment (0, absent; 1, present).

18. Incoherent: Normal grammatical sentence construction has broken down, includes "word salad" and should only be rated conservatively for extreme forms of formal thought disorder (0, absent; 1, present).

19. Positive formal thought disorder: Patient has fluent speech but tends to communicate poorly due to neologisms, bizarre use of words, derailments, or loosening of associations (0, absent; 1, present).

20. Negative formal thought disorder: Includes paucity of thought, frequent thought blocking, poverty of speech, or poverty of content of speech (0, absent; 1, present).

21. Affective symptoms predominate: Depressive or manic features form a prominent part of the illness, and mood disorder alone might explain much or all of the symptoms. Isolated examples of depressed or exalted mood during the course of the illness should not be rated positively for this item. Rate conservatively, as this is an exclusion item for several operational systems for schizophrenia, although it would be present in cases of schizoaffective disorder (0, absent; 1, present).

22. Restricted affect: Patient's emotional responses are restricted in range, and at interview there is an impression of bland indifference of "lack of contact" (0, absent; 1, present).

23. Blunted affect: Where the patient's emotional responses are persistently flat and show a complete failure to "resonate" to external change. The difference between restricted and blunted affect should be regarding as one of degree, with "blunted" only being rated in extreme cases (0, absent; 1, present).

24. Inappropriate affect: Patient's emotional responses are inappropriate to the circumstance, e.g. laughter when discussing painful or sad occurrences, fatuous giggling without apparent reason (0, absent; 1, present).

25. Rapport difficult: Interviewer finds difficulty in establishing contact with the patient, who appears remote or cut off; does not include patients who are difficult to interview because of hostility or irritability (0, absent; 1, present).

26. Persecutory delusions: Includes all delusions with persecutory ideation (0, absent; 1, present)/

27. Well-organised delusions: Illness is characterised by a series of well organised or well-systematised delusions (0, absent; 1, present).

28. Grandiose delusions: Patient has grossly exaggerated sense of his or her own importance, has exceptional abilities, or believes that he or she is rich or famous, titled, or related to royalty. Also included are delusions of identification with God, angels, the Messiah, etc. (see also item 56). (Any duration, score 1; if symptom lasts at least 2 weeks, score 2.).

29. Delusions of influence: Events, objects, or other people in the patient's immediate surroundings have a special significance, often of a persecutory nature; includes ideas of reference from the television, radio, or newspapers, where the patient believes that these are providing instructions or prescribing certain behaviour (0, absent; 1, present).

30. Bizarre delusions: Strange, absurd, or fantastic delusions whose content may have a mystical, magical , or "science fiction" quality (0, absent; 1, present).

31. Widespread delusions: Delusions that intrude into most aspects of the patient's life and/or preoccupy the patient for most of his or her time (0, absent; 1, present).

32. Delusions of passivity: Include all "made" sensations, emotions, or actions. Score 1 for all experiences of influence where the patient knows that his or her own thoughts, feelings, impulses, volitional acts, or somatic sensations are controlled or imposed by an external agency. Score 2 when there are "experiences of alienation", i.e. the patients is aware that thoughts, feelings, etc are not his or her own but are coming from an outside source (0, absent; 1, present).

33. Primary delusional perception: Score 1 where the patient perceives something in the outside world that triggers a special, significant, relatively non-understandable belief of which he or she is certain and that is in some way loosely linked to the triggering perception. Score 2 when the special significance is attached to the perception itself and not merely linked to it (0, absent; 1, present).

34. Other primary delusions: Includes delusional mood and delusional ideas. Delusional mood is.a strange mood in which the environment appears changed in a threatening way but the significance of the change cannot be understood by the patient, who is usually tense, anxious, or bewildered. This can lead to a delusional belief. A delusional idea appears abruptly in the patient's mind fully developed and unheralded by any related thoughts (0, absent; 1, present).

35. Delusions and hallucinations lasting for 1 week: Any type of delusion accompanied by hallucinations of any type lasting 1 week (0, absent; 1, present).

36. Persecutory or jealous content delusions accompanied by hallucinations of any type: this is self-explanatory, but note that abnormal beliefs are of delusional intensity and quality and are accompanied by true hallucinations (0, absent; 1, present).

37. Thought insertion: Score 1 when the patient recognises that thoughts are being put into his or her head that are not the patient's own. Score 2 when the patient experiences thoughts that are not his or her own and have been imposed by an outside agency.

38. Thought withdrawal: Score 1 when the patient experiences thoughts ceasing in his or her head and may experience "pure thought block". Score 2 when the patient experiences an external agency removing thoughts from his or her head.

39. Thought broadcast: Score 1 when the patient experiences thoughts diffusing out of his or her head. Score 2 when the patient experiences thoughts diffusing out of his or her head and they are shared with others, i.e. the belief that others actually hear the thoughts.

40. Thought echo: Score 1 if the patient experiences thoughts repeated or echoed in his or her head. Score 2 if thoughts are repeated by a voice outside the patient's head.

41. Third person auditory hallucinations: Two or more voices discussing the patient in the third person. Score 1 if either "true" or "pseudo" hallucinations, i.e. differentiation of the source of the voices is unimportant. Score 2 if "true" hallucinations can be established, i.e. definitely perceived to arise outside patient's subjective space.

42. Running commentary voices: Patient hears voices describing his or her actions, sensations, or emotions as they occur. Score 1 if there are possible "pseudo" hallucinations, but score 2 if definite "true" hallucinations can be defined (see also definitions of item 41).

43. Abusive/accusatory/persecutory voices: Voices talking to the patient in an accusatory, abusive, or persecutory manner (0, absent; 1, present).

44. Other (non affective) auditory hallucinations: Any other kind of auditory hallucinations; includes pleasant or neutral voices and non verbal hallucinations (0, absent; 1, present).

45.   Information not credible: Patient gives misleading answers to questions and provides a jumbled, incoherent or inconsistent account (0, absent; 1, present).

46.   Lack of insight: Patient is unable to recognise that his or her experiences are abnormal or that they are the produce of an anomalous mental process, or recognises that the experiences are abnormal but gives a delusional explanation (1 indicates lack of insight; 0, insight present).

47.   Deterioration from premorbid level of functioning: Patient does not regain premorbid social, occupational, or emotional functioning after an acute episode of illness (0, absent; 1, deterioration present).

48.   Schizophrenic symptoms respond to neuroleptics: Rate globally over the total period. Score positively if illness appears to respond to any type of neuroleptics (depot or oral) or if relapse occurs when medication is stopped (0, symptoms do not respond; 1, symptoms respond).

49.   Non-affective hallucination: Hallucinations in any modality in which the content has not apparent relationship to elation or depression. Score positively only if they are present throughout the day for several days or intermittently for 1 week (0, absent; 1, present).

50.   Elevated mood: Patient's predominant mood is one of elation lasting at least 1 week to score 1 week to score 1 or lasting at least 2 weeks to score 2. If elation lasted less than 1 week but the patient was hospitalised for affective disorder, score 1.

51.   Irritable mood: Patient's mood is predominantly irritable and lasts at least 1 week to score 1 or at least 2 weeks to score 2. If the patient is hospitalised for affective disorder but less than 1 week of irritable mood, score 1.

52.   Schizophrenic symptoms occur at the same time as affective symptoms: Score positively if dubiety is present whether episode is one of affective disorder or schizophrenia (0, absent; 1, present).

53.   Excessive activity: Patient is markedly overactive. This includes motor, social, and sexual activity. Score 1 for hyperactivity lasting 1 week and 2 for a duration of 2 weeks.

54.   Reckless activity: Patient is excessively involved in activities with high potential for painful consequences that are not recognised, e.g. excessive spending, sexual indiscretions, reckless driving, etc. Duration of 1 week is scored 1, and duration of 2 weeks is scored 2.

55.   Pressured speech: Patient is much more talkative than usual or feels under pressure to continue talking; includes manic type of formal thought disorder with clang associations, punning and rhyming, etc. Score 1 for duration of 1 week and 2 for duration of 2 weeks.

56. Increased self esteem: Patient believes that he or she is an exceptional person with special powers, plans, talents, or abilities. Rate positively here if over valued idea, but if delusional in quality also score item 28 (grandiose delusions). Score 1 if duration is 1 week and 2 if it lasts 2 weeks.

57. Thoughts racing: Patient experiences thoughts racing through his or her head or others observe flights of ideas and find difficulty in following what the patient is saying or in interrupting because of the rapidity and quantity of speech. Duration of 1 week scores 1, and duration of 2 weeks scores 2.

58. Distractibility: Patient experiences difficulty concentrating on what is going on around him or her because attention is too easily drawn to irrelevant or extraneous factors. Duration of 1 week scores 1 and 2 weeks scores 2.

59. Reduced for need for sleep: Patient sleeps less but there is no complaint of insomnia. Extra waking time is usually taken up with excessive activities. Duration of 1 week scores 1 and 2 weeks scores 2.

60. Dysphoria: Persistently low or depressed mood, irritable and sad mood, or pervasive loss of interest. Score 1 if present for at least 1 week, 2 if present for 2 weeks, and 3 if present for 1 month.

61. Agitated activity: Patient shows excessive repetitive activity, such as fidgeting restlessness, wringing of hands, or pacing up and down, all usually accompanied by expression of mental anguish. Score 1 if present for 1 week, 2 if present for 2 weeks, and 3 if present for 1 month.

62. Slowed activity: Patient complains that he or she feels slowed and unable to moved. Others may report a subjective feeling of retardation, or retardation may be noted by the examining clinician. Score 1 if present for 1 week, 2 if present for 2 weeks, and 3 if present for 1 month.

63. Loss of energy/tiredness: Subjective complaints of being excessively tired with no energy. Score 1 for duration of 1 week, 2 for 2 weeks, and 3 for 1 month.

64. Loss of pleasure: Pervasive inability to enjoy any activity. This includes marked loss of interest or loss of libido. Score 1 for duration of 1 week, 2 for 2 weeks, and 3 for 1 month.

65. Poor concentration: Subjective complaint of being unable to think clearly, make decisions, etc. Score 1 for duration of 1 week, 2 for 2 weeks, and 3 for 1 month.

66. Excessive self-reproach: Extreme feelings of guilt and unworthiness. This may be of delusional intensity ("worst person in the whole world"). Score 1 for duration of 1 week, 2 for 2 weeks, and 3 for 1 month.

67. Suicidal ideation: Preoccupation with thoughts of death (not necessarily own); includes thinking of suicide, wishing to be dead, and attempts to kill self. Score 1 for duration of 1 week, 2 for 2 weeks, and 3 for 1 month.

68. Initial insomnia: Patient complains of being unable to get to sleep and lies awake for at least 1 hour. Score 1 for duration of 1 week, 2 for 2 weeks, and 3 for 1 month.

69. Early morning waking: Patient complains of persistently waking up at least 1 hour earlier than usual waking time. Score 1 for duration of 1 week, 2 for 2 weeks, and 3 for 1 month.

70. Excessive sleep: Patient complains of sleeping too much. Score 1 if present for 1 week, 2 for 2 weeks, and 3 for 1 month.

71. Poor appetite: Subjective complaint that the patient has a poor appetite (not necessarily observed to be eating less). Score 1 if present for 1 week, 2 for 2 weeks, and 3 for 1 month.

72. Weight loss: Weight loss of at least 0.9 kg per week or 4.5 kg per year when not dieting. Score 1 for duration one week, 2 for 2 weeks, and 3 for 1 month.

73. Increased appetite: Patient reported increased appetite and/or comfort eating. Score 1 for duration of 1 week, 2 for 2 weeks, and 3 for 1 month.

74. Weight gain: Weight gain of at least 0.9 kg per week or 4.5 kg per year. Score 1 for duration of 1 week, 2 for 2 weeks, and 3 for 1 month.

Author index

Subject index

For Product Safety Concerns and Information please contact our EU
representative GPSR@taylorandfrancis.com
Taylor & Francis Verlag GmbH, Kaufingerstraße 24, 80331 München, Germany

www.ingramcontent.com/pod-product-compliance
Ingram Content Group UK Ltd.
Pitfield, Milton Keynes, MK11 3LW, UK
UKHW021440080625
459435UK00011B/320